SHORT NOTES FOR THE DCH

SHORT NOTES FOR THE DCH

Joseph Blackburn
MA BM BCh MRCP MRCGP DRCOG DCH

Graham Curtis Jenkins
MA MB BChir FRCGP DRCOG

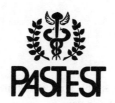

PASTEST

© 1990 PasTest
Rankin House,
Parkgate Estate,
Knutsford, Cheshire, WA16 8DX, England.

First published 1990
Reprinted 1992
Revised edition 1994

British Library Cataloguing in Publication Data
Blackburn J.
>Short Notes for the DCH (Diploma in Child Health)
>1. Paediatrics
>I. Title II. Curtis-Jenkins, G.
>618.92

ISBN: 0 - 906896 - 29 - 0

Text prepared and lasertypeset by Dr J Blackburn.
Printed by BPCC Wheatons, Exeter.

CONTENTS

USER GUIDE

This is not a textbook - it is a course of study that will enable you to pass the Diploma in Child Health (DCH). A second edition has allowed us to remain up-to-date on topics such as childhood immunisations and the law relating to children which have changed dramatically since 1990.

This book contains:

- A study guide for the DCH examination.
- Model answers for the 'Short Note Questions' of Paper I.
- Synopses of topics that commonly arise in the 'Case Commentary Questions' of Paper I and the clinical examination.
- The type of information examined by the multiple choice questions in Paper II.

In general, chapters are arranged by *specialty* and divided into *symptoms*. The information is presented as notes. Duplication has been minimised. For example, the main description of Henoch Schonlein Purpura appears in the Haematology section but the renal involvement is mentioned in the Urinary Tract section.

You will see rare conditions mentioned as causes of common symptoms. Unless these conditions are likely to turn up in the examination we have not described them in detail.

We recommend that you start by reading through this book once. Then take a section at a time and make your own notes for each heading. You will find any further information you need among the short list of books in the bibliography. Update your notes if you see an interesting review article in a journal. This helps to consolidate the information in your memory.

One of us (GCJ) has been an examiner for the DCH and is acknowledged as an authority on paediatric care in general practice; the other (JB) would claim to be an expert at passing examinations. We hope that our book will pass our knowledge on to you.

Dedication

I would like to dedicate this book to my children, Julia and Claire Blackburn, who forgave me when I deserted them in order to sit in front of my word processor. This book would not have even been conceived if they had not taught me the reality of 'child health'.

ABBREVIATIONS

Ab	Antibody.
Ag	Antigen.
ASOT	Anti-Streptolysin O Titre.
CAH	Congenital Adrenal Hyperplasia.
CxR	Chest X-Ray.
ECG	Electro-Cardiogram.
EEG	Electro-Encephalogram.
EMG	Electro-Myelogram.
ESR	Erythrocyte Sedimentation Rate.
FBC	Full Blood Count.
G6PDH	Glucose 6-Phosphate Dehydrogenase.
HIV	Human Immune Deficiency Virus.
HOCM	Hypertrophic Obstructive Cardiomyopathy.
i.v.	intravenous.
IVP	Intravenous Pyelogram.
IVU	Intravenous Urogram.
JCA	Juvenile Chronic Arthritis.
NSAID	Non-Steroidal Anti-Inflammatory Drugs.
PKU	Phenylketonuria.
RBC	Red Blood Cell.
SBE	Subacute Bacterial Endocarditis.
SLE	Systemic Lupus Erythematosis.
SSPE	Subacute Sclerosing Panencephalitis.
USS	Ultrasound Scan.
UTI	Urinary Tract Infection.
WBC	White Blood Cell.
VSD	Ventricular Septal Defect.

BIBLIOGRAPHY

Treatment and Prognosis: Paediatrics. Editors G. Clayden and R. Hawkins. Heinemann Medical Books (1988).

Textbook of Paediatrics. Editors J.O. Forfar and G.C. Arneil. Churchill Livingstone (1984).

Child Care in General Practice. Editors C. Hart and John Bain. Churchill Livingstone (1989).

Community Paediatrics. Editors D. Hull and L. Polnay. Churchill Livingstone (1985).

The Development of the Infant and Young Child. R.S. Illingworth. Churchill Livingstone (1980).

Immunisation against Infectious Disease. Editors D. Salisbury and N. Begg. HMSO (1992)

1. DEMOGRAPHIC STATISTICS

The following statistics are derived from the annual reports of the Office of Population Censuses and Surveys which are published by Her Majesty's Stationery Office (HMSO).

STILL BIRTH RATE
= the number of still births per 1000 total births
Incidence. Stable at 6 from 1983 to 1986.
Significance. Reflects social and economic factors more than obstetric care. Doubles from social class I to V. 60% of stillbirths are due to abnormalities of the placenta or umbilical cord, toxaemia, and other maternal disese. 40% of stillbirths are due to fetal disease or abnormality. Complications of the delivery such as trauma and hypoxia account for 10% of these stillbirths.

INFANT MORTALITY
= deaths within 1 year of birth per 1000 live births
Incidence. Fell from 12 in 1980 to 9.1 in 1985.
Significance. The infant mortality rate (IMR) is a very crude measure of the effectiveness of health care provision. In developed nations a significant proportion of such deaths is associated with congenital malformations incompatible with life and sudden infant deaths. However, given this limitation the UK has one of the highest rates in Western Europe. The IMR varies with the social class of the mother: Relative Risk for Social class I = 1; II and III (non-manual) = 1.1; IV (manual) = 1.6; V = 2.2. The IMR is higher for illegitimate births and children born to teenage mothers. The IMR increases from South to North across the UK.

NEONATAL MORTALITY
= deaths between birth and day 27 per 1000 live births
Incidence. Fell from 7.6 in 1980 to 5.3 in 1985.
Significance. See perinatal mortality.

EARLY NEONATAL MORTALITY
= deaths in the first week of life per 1000 live births
Incidence. 2.1 in 1983, 1.9 in 1986.
Significance. See perinatal mortality.

LATE NEONATAL MORTALITY
= neonatal deaths occurring after the first week per 1000 live births
Incidence. 1.2 in 1983, 1.0 in 1986.

1

PERINATAL MORTALITY
= still births + early neonatal mortality per 1000 births
Incidence. Stable at 7.9.
Significance. Low birth weight, prematurity, congenital abnormality and perinatal hypoxia account for most cases of perinatal death. Improved obstetric care would scarcely dent the incidence of perinatal mortality.

POST NEONATAL MORTALITY
= deaths between 28 days and 1 year per 1000 live births
Incidence. No significant improvement from 4.2 in 1983.
Significance. Lower social class, illegitimacy, large families and winter are associated with an increased post neonatal mortality. The common causes are respiratory infections (30%), sudden infant death syndrome (25%), congenital heart disease (10%), and accidents (5%).

MORTALITY RATE IN CHILDHOOD AFTER INFANCY
= deaths between age 1 and 14 per 1000 children aged 1 to 14
Incidence. 3.4 per 1000 children aged 1 to 14.
Significance. Mortality rates fall progressively after infancy. The commonest causes of death are accidents and respiratory diseases. Meningitis, neoplasia and congenital heart disease are less common but concern more parents.

MORBIDITY
The majority, probably 90%, of childhood illnesses are cared for by parents without the advice of a doctor. Of those conditions that present to General Practitioners the majority are due to infections or trauma. About 10% of consultations result in a referral to a specialist. Each year 10% of children are admitted to hospital.

DISABILITY AND HANDICAP
Disability is the loss or reduction of functional capacity. Handicap is the disadvantage or restriction of activity caused by a disability. Hence, paralysis of the legs is a disability. The corresponding handicap is limited mobility. Wheelchairs and ramps reduce the handicap without affecting the disability. Around 0.7% of children suffer from severe physical or mental handicaps. 7% have a less severe chronic disability or illness. A concise review of the medical and social implications of a disability is found in chapter 40 of 'Child Care in General Practice'.

2. SUDDEN DEATH

EPIDEMIOLOGY
Twice as many children die before age 1 as die after. The common causes of
death before age 1 are, in order of importance, perinatal disorders, congenital
anomalies, respiratory tract infections, sudden infant death syndrome, and
neoplasms. After age 1 the common causes are accidents, infections
(respiratory>meningitis and enteritis), neoplasms, congenital anomalies,
respiratory disease and violence.

MANAGEMENT OF SUDDEN DEATH
A child who dies suddenly is usually taken to hospital by his parents in the
hope that he can be resuscitated. The GP should visit the parents as soon as he
hears of the death. Occasionally a GP is called to see a child who has died at
home. If there is no possibility of successful resuscitation:
• Call the coroner's officer who will tell the parents of the required legal
  process and arrange for the body to be taken to a mortuary.
• Discuss the death with the parents (and the siblings if appropriate). A
  sedative may be needed in order to permit some sleep. Suppress lactation.
  Arrange to visit again after the post-mortem examination.
• On the next visit discuss the results of the post-mortem. Discuss the risk
  of other children being affected. Provide information leaflets and the contact
  number for a relevant support group.
• Monitor the grieving process in the family members. The health visitor is
  often well suited to this role.

SUDDEN INFANT DEATH SYNDROME
A sudden and unexpected death that cannot be adequately explained by the
findings on necropsy.
Aetiology. Probably multifactorial. Possibly hyperthermia due to
overwrapping during an infection (2/3 have signs of gastroenteritis or
respiratory infection on the day of death). Possibly idiopathic or obstructive
apnoea. A few may represent non-accidental injury.
Incidence. 3/1000 live births (20% of infant deaths). Commonest at 3
months (1-6 months). Commoner in winter and in cities. UK has 4 times the
rate in Sweden.
Risk factors. No association with bottle feeding or difficult delivery.
• Mother aged <25, unmarried, immigrant, socio-economic class V.
• Narcotic addict (x30)
• Risk increases with parity, especially if pregnancies come close together.
• Previous child died with SIDS (x10).
• Baby is a twin, low birth weight, had apnoeic episodes.

Management. Increased social support to families at risk and apnoea alarms do not prevent SID.

ACCIDENTS

Incidence. Accidents are the largest single cause of death in childhood (age 1–15). One third of childhood deaths are due to accidents. Each day 3 children die in accidents in Britain. Each year 10% of children attend a doctor because of an accidental injury. Boys of social classes IV and V are at greatest risk. About 1% of chronic handicap in childood is due to accidents, especially head injuries.

Aetiology.

- Road accidents (50% of deaths). A car hitting a child pedestrian or cyclist is the commonest fatal accident in childhood.
- Accident at home (30% of deaths). Falls are the commonest accident, scalds and burns are the commonest lethal accident in the home, choking on inhaled foreign bodies, suffocation by plastic.
- Accidents outside the home (20% of deaths): falls, drowning.

Prevention.

- Primary prevention: education (road safety); legislation or regulation (speed limits); design (pedestrian crossings and anti-lock brakes), maintenance (of cars). Some families seem accident prone. This may reflect an inability to perceive dangers, a disorganised lifestyle or neglect. In practice it is difficult to influence dangerous patterns of behaviour or teach a parent how to identify dangers.
- Secondary prevention: seat belts.
- Tertiary prevention: teaching parents first aid.

Treatment. Ensure that you are familiar with the management of:

- Common fractures and injuries to the head, abdomen and spine.
- Scalds and burns.
- Inhaled foreign bodies and drowning.

POISONING

Incidence. Each year in Britain 40,000 children attend casualty with suspected poisoning, 11,000 are admitted but only 20 die. Age 1-5 years.

- Medicines are taken accidentally by children. Adolescents may take intentional overdoses.
- Household products such as bleaches.
- Plant berries.

Prevention. Child resistant caps on medicine bottles (standard since 1989). Lock up medicines and cleaning agents.

Treatment. A child who has ingested a potentially toxic substance should be taken to hospital immediately. Ensure that you are familiar with the management of poisoning with: paracetamol, aspirin, tricyclic antidepressants, bleach, organic solvents, iron.

NON-ACCIDENTAL INJURY

Incidence. 5,000 children each year are recognized as seriously abused. 500 die.

Risk factors.
- Child < 3 years old (cannot complain and needs more care).
- The child is unwanted (illegitimate, step-child).
- The child is difficult to look after (congenitally abnormal, sick, born prematurely).
- The child or a sibling was previously battered,
- The abusing parent was abused.
- The abusing parent generally has difficulty coping with life (young, social class V, psychiatric problems).

Clinically.
- Violence, sexual abuse, emotional abuse. Presents with an injury, behaviour problems, or learning difficulties.
- Physical or emotional neglect. Presents with failure to thrive.

Management. A GP who suspects abuse might refer the child to:
- A paediatrician (to exclude physical illnesses that can mimic abuse, and look for positive evidence of abuse).
- A social worker (to remove the child and siblings to a place of safety, to support the family, to call a case conference).
- Others: teachers, health visitors, police.

A case conference is an opportunity to share information and plan action (nothing, key worker, "At-risk" register, family therapy, police prosecution, care proceedings). The legal implications of child abuse are set out in chapter 3.

Prognosis. 25% will be abused again.

3. LAW

REGISTRATION OF BIRTH
- Within 42 days of delivery.
- Registered by anyone present at the birth.

REGISTRATION OF STILLBIRTH
- No sign of life when delivered after the 28th week of pregnancy.
- Registered by midwife or doctor attending birth.

DEFINITIONS OF CHILDHOOD
The protection offered to a child and the expected degree of personal responsibility is related to age.
- A child is a person under 18 years old for inheritance, marriage without parental consent and the right to vote.
- Heterosexual intercourse and marriage with parent's consent is legal from age 16. It is illegal for a man to have intercourse with a girl under 16 years old (unless she is more than 13 years old, he is under 24 years old, and he believed her to be over 16 years old).
- In criminal law. A child under age 10 cannot be held responsible for a crime, but can be placed in local authority (LA) care for 'care and control'. For a child aged 10 to 14 the prosecution must show that a child was aware that he was doing wrong. A child under 14 years cannot be prosecuted for rape. A 'young person' aged 14 to 16 years old is assumed to be aware he was doing wrong unless this can be disproved. A young person may appear in a special 'juvenile court' but a 17 year old can be prosecuted in an ordinary court. A child or young person charged with a grave crime (murder) can be tried in a crown court.

EDUCATION
Under the Education Act 1944 every child over 5 years old and under the school leaving age must receive full time education. The school leaving age is the end of the spring or summer term next following the child's 16th birthday. A child need not attend school if his parents can prove that he is receiving an adequate education at home.

DAILY CHILD CARE
The Nurseries and Child-Minders Regulation Act 1948 made LAs responsible for regulating daily minding in private homes and other places (nurseries etc). Child-minder and premises must be approved by the LA if children are looked after for more than 2 hours each day. In 1991 the Children Act 1989 extended the regulations to children up to age 8 years.

CONSENT TO MEDICAL CARE

A person over age 16 can legally give his own consent. Below age 16, the consent of his parent or guardian is required unless:

- Emergency treatment is required. Consent by a person such as a teacher who is *in loco parentis* is only applicable to an emergency for which such consent is unnecessary.
- The child has given consent **and** the doctor considers that the child is of sufficient understanding to make an informed decision about medical care (including contraception) **and** the child will not agree to a parent being asked for consent.

If a child under age 16 refuses consent, a doctor cannot proceed (even if the child is under a care order etc) unless:

- he believes that the child does not have sufficient understanding to make an informed decision.
- a court has considered the child's objection and told the doctor to proceed.

If the parent(s) of a child under age 16 refuse a life-saving treatment, a court can give consent.

CONFIDENTIALITY

- A person aged 16 has full rights to confidentiality.
- Under age 16, a doctor may generally divulge information to parents without the child's permission. However, a child has a right to confidentiality if a doctor has judged him capable of giving informed consent.
- If a doctor suspects that the child is subject to severe physical or sexual abuse he should discuss the situation with his medical defence association who would generally advise him to inform the local authority.
- A doctor may break confidentiality to release information to police investigating a grave or serious crime.

PARENTAL RIGHTS

- A mother and father have equal parental rights and responsibilities for a legitimate child.
- An unmarried father is financially responsible for his child but has no intrinsic rights.
- Step-parents have no legal rights, but they have financial responsibilities towards a step-child.
- Adopting parents are the sole legal parents.

- When a child is made a ward of the High Court, all major decisions (sterilisation, abortion) must be decided by the court until the child is 18 or the order is discharged. Anyone can request wardship proceedings, but the LA can stop the application. Since 1991, wardship has been reserved for extreme cases.

ADOPTION
In 1984 9,000 children were adopted. Half were illegitimate.
- The adopted child has no claim to maintenance or inheritance from his original parent(s). He takes on the nationality of his adoptive parents.
- Adoption is arranged by registered agencies (charities, local authorities) or relatives. Applicants must be aged 21 or more. Adoption orders can be made in a magistrates court, high court or county court.
- A reporting officer is appointed to ensure that the natural parents give informed consent. If the child is illegitimate, only the mother's consent is needed. The parents' consent is not needed if they cannot be found, are incapable of agreeing, have abandoned or neglected the child, have persistently ill-treated the child and are unlikely to ever be able to look after the child adequately.
- The child must live with the adoptive parents for three months before the order is finalised.
- All rights and responsibilities pass to the adoptive parents irreversibly. The original parents have no right of access.
- At age 18 an adopted child is entitled to his original birth certificate.

CHILD PROTECTION

Child destruction
The Infant Life Preservation Act (1929) made it illegal to cause the death of any unborn child over 28 weeks gestation except to preserve the mother's life.
Infanticide
A woman who causes the death of her infant by wilful act or omission is guilty of a lesser crime than murder if the balance of her mind was disturbed by childbirth or lactation.
Child abuse
In common law every parent and any person who looks after another's child has a duty to exercise reasonable care. The Children and Young Persons Act 1933 made it a crime to assault, ill-treat, neglect, abandon or expose a child. Neglect includes not providing adequate food, clothing, medical aid or lodging.

The Children Act 1989
The Act took effect in October 1991. It is based on the following principles:
- The welfare of the child is the paramount consideration of the court.
- The child's wishes must be considered in matters affecting his welfare. A child, although too young to understand the oath, may give evidence.
- The court must consider the child's race, religion, culture and language.
- A court should not make an order if the child would be better cared for in the absence of a court order.
- Parental responsibility replaces the concept of parental rights.
- A child should remain with his family whenever possible.

Private law cases involving disputes between individuals with parental responsibility are settled in a county court by judges.
- A Contact Order determines who should have access to a child.
- A Residence Order defines where a child will live.
- A Prohibited Steps Order prohibits an action such as taking a child abroad.
- A Specific Issue Order rules on any other issue such as choice of school.
- A Parental Responsibility Order allows an unmarried father to apply for parental rights denied him by the child's mother.

Children and families in need
Social Services must provide support to enable families to care for their children. Services commonly provided include:
- Guidance by an assigned social worker or a worker in a family centre.
- Financial assistance and accommodation.
- Family aides to help with child care, cooking, cleaning and washing.
- Daycare with a child-minder, playgroup or nursery.
- Youth clubs and holiday outings for older children.
- Respite care for children with disabilities to allow parents a rest.

When LAs agree to a parent's request that their child be placed in voluntary accommodation away from home:
- The LA must ensure that a good standard of care is provided.
- Parents may take their child home at any time.
- The child should be placed as near to the family home as possible.
- The child should be placed with relatives or friends of the family if possible.
- Children of the same family should usually be kept together.
- The LA must encourage regular contact between children and their families.
LAs should only seek a court order when all else has failed.

9

Public law cases including children who are beyond the control of their parent(s) and children in danger usually come before a magistrate in a Family Proceedings Court. A few of the more serious cases are transferred to the county court or High Court.

Parents rights in public law cases include:
- Immediate legal aid without a means test.
- To be informed about any action being taken that concerns their child. They should be told in advance unless the situation is so serious that the LA must act immediately.
- To put their case in court.
- To be involved in deciding how their child is looked after by a LA even if their child has been taken into care under a court order.

The child's interests are usually represented by a social worker appointed by the court and independent of the LA, called a *guardian ad litem*.

When there is reasonable cause to suspect that a child is suffering, or is likely to suffer significant harm the Children Act offers the following remedies:
- A Supervision Order requires parents to permit a probation officer or an officer of the LA to see their child. Lasts 1 year unless extended.
- An Education Supervision Order allows the LA to supervise a child's education. Lasts 1 year unless extended.
- A Child Assessment Order (CAO) directs a parent to allow their child to be assessed for up to 7 days. This may include removal from the family home.
- The Emergency Protection Order (EPO) lasts 8 days and can be extended for another 7 days. Applications may be made by any person. The court may direct the police to enter premises to enforce the order, and may specify where the child is to be held and any medical or other assessments required.
- The Police Protection Order allows the police to remove and hold a child for up to 72 hours.
- A Recovery Order requires the police to find a child who has been unlawfully taken away or has run away. The police have the power to enter premises to search for the child.
- A Care Order gives the LA parental responsibility until the child is aged 18. The local authority may not change the child's name or religion, and cannot offer the child for adoption.
- A Secure Accommodation Order allows a LA to confine a child in order to protect the child or prevent the child from hurting other people.
- A Family Assistance Order requires a LA or court welfare officer to give a family help and support. The court uses this order at its own discretion – it cannot be applied for.

4. ANTENATAL CARE

PRE-CONCEPTION COUNSELLING
- **Spacing pregnancies.** Pregnancy is safest and the perinatal mortality is lowest when the birth interval is 18 to 48 months. There is an increased miscarriage rate if conception occurs immediately on stopping the contraceptive pill.
- **Weight.** An underweight mother is more likely to deliver a low birth weight baby.
- **Vitamins.** Women who have had a baby with a neural tube defect may reduce the risk in subsequent pregnancies by taking B vitamins prior to conception.
- **Infections.** Check rubella status. High vaginal swab if symptomatic.
- **Drugs.** Prescribed medication should be rationalised to minimise the risk to the fetus. Chronic diseases such as diabetes and hypertension should be well controlled prior to any attempt at conception. Drugs of addiction (tobacco, alcohol, heroin) should be avoided.
- **Genetic counselling.** See the chapter on genetic abnormalities.

ADVICE DURING PREGNANCY
- **Sport.** Strenuous exertion might impair placental function.
- **Sex.** Intercourse should be avoided for at least 1 week after vaginal bleeding in pregnancy. Multiple sexual partners increase the risk of contracting infections that might damage the fetus.
- **Work.** Physically exhausting work might impair placental function in the last trimester. Sedentary jobs can be continued up to the day of delivery.
- **Diet.** Excessive weight gain or loss should be avoided.

HIGH RISK PREGNANCIES
Factors recognized at booking
1. Familial conditions.
2. Maternal factors.
   - Old or young.
   - Short (under 5 feet tall), underweight, small or malformed pelvis.
   - Poor obstetric history and infertility.
   - Multiparity is only associated with a worse outcome if there were problems with previous pregnancies.
   - Low socio-economic class, late booking and failure to attend for antenatal care are associated with increased perinatal mortality.
   - Maternal nutrition: vegan.
   - Drugs: prescribed, over-the-counter (tobacco, alcohol), and illicit.
   - Maternal illness: SLE, diabetes, Grave's disease, infections.

Factors developing during the pregnancy
- Severe anaemia (<9 g/dl), gestational diabetes, pre-eclampsia.
- Maternal infections: urinary tract infection, rubella, cytomegalovirus, toxoplasmosis, Listeria monocytogenes, syphilis, human immune deficiency virus, vaginal herpes simplex.
- Rhesus iso-immunisation.
- Threatened miscarriage, placental abruption, intrauterine growth retardation.
- Twins, malpresentation, hydramnios, oligohydramnios.
- Premature labour or premature rupture of membranes.
- Post-term.

ROUTINE MONITORING
- Booking blood tests: Hb, Rhesus abs, VDRL, rubella titre, (HIV).
- Infection screen: vaginal swabs and urine cultures as indicated.
- Regular assessment of weight, blood pressure, uterine size, proteinuria and glycosuria. After 30 weeks: fetal presentation, movements and heart rate.
- Ultrasound for fetal size and growth. Major congenital malformations can be identified by 19 weeks gestation.

SPECIAL ASSESSMENT OF FETAL STATUS
- Ultrasound. Fetal movements and growth reflect fetal health towards term.
- The level of fetal products in maternal urine or blood (oestriol, human placental lactogen) usually rises during pregnancy. A fall or a failure to rise is a better predictor of fetal well-being than the absolute level.
- Amniotic fluid analysis for genetic abnormalities and neural tube defects, fetal age and pulmonary maturation.
- Cardiotocograph (CTG): Fetal death is uncommon in the 48 hours after a normal fetal heart record.

MEDICAL INTERVENTION DURING PREGNANCY
- Parentcraft classes.
- Treat maternal disease avoiding feto-toxic medication.
- Treat Rhesus iso-immunisation.
- Antenatal diagnosis of abnormalities with therapeutic abortion.
- Inhibit premature labour.
- Elective caesarean section.
- Induce post-term pregnancies (to avoid placental insufficiency).
- Active management to prevent long labours. Intrapartum monitoring to detect fetal hypoxia (CTG, scalp vein pH).
- Paediatric staff available at deliveries. Special care baby units.

5. THE NEONATE

THE NORMAL NEONATE

ROUTINE CARE
- At birth the nasopharynx is cleared with a mucus extractor, the cord is clamped (Hollister clamp), and the baby is given to the mother to cuddle and dry. The neonate is taken to be weighed, measured and examined. Vitamin K is given intramuscularly to prevent haemorrhagic disease of the newborn (1/400 live births).
- The baby is fed as soon as the mother feels able, and on demand thereafter.
- Urine should be passed within 24 hours and meconium within 48 hours.
- Daily care during the first 10 days includes: cleaning the cord stump, weighing, and monitoring for infection.
- On day 7 capillary blood is tested for phenylalanine (Guthrie test) and thyroid stimulating hormone.

EXAMINATION OF THE NEWBORN
Consider risk factors (social, familial, antenatal, intra-partum, postnatal).
- General appearance, limb deformities, spine, fontanelle, rashes.
- Responsiveness to faces, noises, light.
- Tone and primitive reflexes (Moro, standing, stepping).
- Head circumference, length and weight.
- Eyes: conjunctivitis, red reflex.
- Mouth and palate.
- Chest: recession, tachypnoea, heart murmur.
- Abdomen: organomegaly, umbilicus, anus, genitals.
- Hips: dislocation, femoral pulses (coarctation), hernias.
- Blood test: PKU, hypothyroidism, haemoglobinopathy.
Take the opportunity to discuss mothercraft.

FEEDING
In early infancy a well fed baby gains 30 grams per day on milk. Solids should not be introduced before 3 months. Unmodified cows' milk should not be introduced before 6 months (risk of hypocalcaemia and hypernatraemia).

Breastfeeding
Colostrum is secreted for 2 days after delivery during which time a breast-fed baby will lose weight and needs 5% dextrose to prevent dehydration. Suckling and emptying the breast promotes milk flow. Once lactation is established the baby will take 50 ml a breast in 5 minutes. Feed on demand. Give vitamin drops until the baby is weaned or starts formula milk.

Bottlefeeding

Formula feeds are modified from cows' milk by adding lactose and vitamins and reducing the content of sodium, phosphate and protein. Initially the baby is fed on demand but within a few weeks most are taking 150 ml/kg/day divided into 3-4 hourly feeds.

Advantages of breastfeeding

- Promotes bonding with the mother.
- The milk is always available.
- The milk is more easily absorbed than cows' milk. The functional importance of this is uncertain.
- Postpones, and may reduce, the risk of cows' milk allergy. May reduce the incidence of eczema in children of atopic parents.
- Difficult to overfeed or prepare the feed incorrectly.
- Less gastroenteritis (antibacterial substances or less contamination).

Advantages of bottlefeeding

- Some women dislike the process of breastfeeding.
- Promotes bonding with the father. He can help with night feeds.
- Feeding in public does not require undressing.
- Allows the mother to return to work sooner after the delivery.

SMALL WORRIES

1. Rashes (see 'birthmarks' in the 'Dermatology' chapter).
2. Regurgitation (see 'vomiting' in 'Gastrointestinal tract').
3. Colic (see 'abdominal pain' in 'Gastrointestinal tract').
4. Crying. Neonates can cry or remain silent. Crying may express the discomfort of a wet nappy, hunger, or boredom. A baby also cries because of pain and disease. Parents vary in how fast they learn to tell the difference.

THE ABNORMAL NEONATE

THE NEONATE AT RISK

- Social, familial and antenatal risk factors (see previous chapter).
- Antenatal complications.
- Low birth weight.
- Complicated delivery.
- Congenital abnormalities.
- Postnatal complications.

LOW BIRTH WEIGHT (LBW)

LBW = liveborn babies weighing less than 2500 grams.
Very LBW = liveborn babies weighing less than 1500 grams.

Incidence. 7% of live born babies are of LBW:

- 5% Premature = less than 37 completed weeks of gestation.
- 2% Small for gestational age. May reflect a defect in the neonate or intrauterine growth retardation (IUGR) due to placental insufficiency or maternal factors (hypertension, smoking, alcohol, undernutrition).
- Both.

Problems of premature neonates.

- Recurrent apnoea.
- Respiratory distress syndrome.
- Starvation. Babies of less than 34 weeks of completed gestation cannot drink enough milk, and need tube or intravenous feeding.
- Dehydration due to a poor fluid intake and/or a high rate of evaporation.
- Hypothermia.
- Jaundice of prematurity.
- Anaemia of prematurity.
- Haemorrhagic disease of the newborn (Vitamin K deficiency).
- Necrotizing enterocolitis.
- Retrolental fibroplasia = proliferative retinopathy. Associated with excessive oxygen therapy (? causally). Affects 20% of LBW neonates but less than 1% become blind. No proven treatment.
- Intraventricular haemorrhage (IVH). 40% of VLBW neonates or babies more than 5 weeks premature. Detected by ultrasound scan. No agreed therapy. Mild IVH does not affect prognosis. Severe IVH kills more than 50% and most of the survivors have hydrocephalus, brain cysts and neurological handicaps.

Problems of small for gestational age (SGA) babies.

- All the problems described for preterm babies.
- Increased incidence of congenital malformations.
- Asphyxia and meconium aspiration.
- Hypoglycaemia. Common during the first 48 hours due to depleted glycogen stores. Causes twitching or seizures. Give oral or i.v. glucose.
- Hypocalcaemia.
- Hypothermia. Neonates, especially LBW, are prone to cooling by evaporation and radiation. The baby is cold, blue, still and oedematous. There is a risk of heart failure on rewarming.
- Polycythaemia, thrombocytopenia and coagulation abnormalities.
- Intrapulmonary haemorrhage.

Prognosis.
- Up to 50% have mental handicap and learning difficulties.
- Remain small.
- Increased incidence of convulsions.

BIRTH TRAUMA
Incidence. Minor injuries are not uncommon.
Aetiology.
- Big baby and small pelvis.
- Twins.
- Abnormal delivery: breach, precipitate delivery of a LBW baby.

Clinically.
- Brain damage or haemorrhage is suggested by an irritable or lethargic baby who feeds poorly. Later signs include vomiting, hypotonia, hypertonia, convulsions, and apnoea.
- Cephalhaematoma, depressed fracture, facial palsy and fat necrosis are external indications of trauma to the head.
- Shoulder injuries include fractured clavicle and brachial plexus stretch. The baby does not move the arm. Usually resolve.

Prognosis. 10% have a continuing handicap. Less than 500 neonates die each year in Britain as a result of birth trauma.

BIRTH ASPHYXIA
Incidence. 2/1,000 live births. At risk: LBW, twins, fetal distress (meconium liquor, bradycardia), difficult delivery (forceps, breech), anaemia.
Clinically. Birth asphyxia = an Apgar score <6 at 5 minutes after delivery. Severe asphyxia = Apgar <3. Seizures are common.

Score	Activity	Pulse	Grimace	Appearance	Respiration
0	Limp	Absent	None	Blue, pale	Absent
1	Some flexion	<100	Grimace	Extremities blue	Slow & irregular
2	Active	>100	Cries	All pink	Good

Investigation. As described for seizures.

Treatment.
- Resuscitate and ventilate.
- Reduce intracranial pressure by restricting fluids, hyperventilation, and i.v. mannitol.

Prognosis. 10% die and 20% of the survivors are handicapped (cerebral palsy, blind, deaf, developmental delay, epilepsy).

BREATHING DIFFICULTIES
- Lung disease.
- Heart failure. See 'Cardiovascular' chapter.
- Neurological disease.

RESPIRATORY DISTRESS
Clinically. Tachypnoea, recession, grunting, central cyanosis. Eventually exhaustion, oedema, shock and episodes of apnoea.
Aetiology.
- Transient tachypnoea syndrome.
- Respiratory distress syndrome (hyaline membrane disease).
- Congenital heart disease.
- Pneumothorax.
- Pneumonia (primary pneumonia or aspiration pneumonia).
- Sepsis.
- Metabolic acidosis.
- Severe anaemia.
- Congenital abnormality of the airways, lungs or chest: airway obstruction, diaphragmatic hernia, hypoplastic lung, congenital lobar emphysema.
- Muscle weakness.

Transient tachypnoea syndrome
Incidence. 10% of live births. Commonest cause of neonatal respiratory distress.
Aetiology. The fetal lung produces fluid to fill the alveoli. Sometimes this continues for up to 48 hours after delivery and causes mild to moderate respiratory distress. CxR shows coarse streakiness and hyperinflation.
Treatment. Oxygen and limited handling.

Respiratory distress syndrome (RDS)
Incidence. 1% of live births. Incidence decreases as gestational age increases. Commonest cause of death in premature babies. Other risk factors: boys, twins, diabetic mother, birth asphyxia, caesarean section, hypothermia.

Aetiology. Inadequate surfactant to keep the alveoli open in expiration.

Clinically. Respiratory distress starts 1-4 hours after delivery, is worst after 2 days and settles a week or two later.

Investigation. A low lecithin/syringomyelin ratio (<2) in amniotic fluid predicts a risk of RDS. The CxR ('ground-glass' with air bronchogram) and blood gases suggest the diagnosis after delivery.

Treatment.

- Prednisolone given to the mother reduces the incidence of RDS in neonates born 24 hours to 7 days after starting treatment. The effect is greatest at 30-34 weeks of gestational age.
- Oxygen, frusemide, nasogastric or i.v. feeding.
- Nebulised surfactant may help.

Prognosis. Overall 10% die and 10% of survivors are neurologically handicapped. Of those requiring ventilation 20% die, and more than 50% develop a serious complication (intraventricular haemorrhage, pneumothorax, emphysema, bronchopulmonary dysplasia, subglottic stenosis, retrolental fibroplasia).

Aspiration

Incidence. 3% of live births.

Aetiology. Meconium > milk, gastric contents.

Clinically. Respiratory distress.

Investigation. CxR shows patchy infiltrates and hyperinflation.

Treatment. Clear nasopharynx and trachea. Some need ventilation.

Prognosis. Good, unless requiring ventilation.

APNOEA AND HYPOVENTILATION

Incidence. 1% of live births have recurrent apnoea (75% of those born at 29 weeks gestation, 7% at 35 weeks gestation).

Clinically. Slow, irregular breathing and episodes of apnoea. Apnoea causes bradycardia,

Aetiology. Prematurity, brain damage, terminal respiratory distress, any serious illness, sedatives given to the mother before delivery.

Treatment.

- Apnoea alarms, gentle stimulation, oxygen, theophylline.
- Some need continuous positive airways pressure (CPAP) or intermittent positive pressure ventilation (IPPV).

Prognosis. Apnoea of prematurity does not increase the risk of mortality or neurological handicap if prolonged apnoea is prevented. The episodes gradually become less frequent and stop at term.

POST–TERM INFANT
= delivery after 42 weeks of gestation.
Clinically. The baby is thin with dry skin.
Complications. Intrauterine death, intrapartum asphyxia or trauma. Aspiration pneumonia.

INFECTIONS
Transplacental infections
Cytomegalovirus and rubella are uncommon, other infections are rare (syphilis, toxoplasmosis, Herpes simplex, Varicella zoster, HIV).
Clinically.
- First trimester: abortion or malformation.
- Second trimester: focal damage or intra-uterine growth retardation (IUGR).
- Third trimester: stillbirth, premature labour, infected neonate.

Intra-partum infections are acquired from infected amniotic fluid or the mother's vagina.
- Streptococcus pyogenes and E. coli cause neonatal pneumonia, septicaemia and meningitis. The fetus is at risk if the membranes rupture more than 24 hours before delivery allowing the liquor to become infected.
- E. coli UTI is commoner in neonates born to mothers with a UTI.
- Herpes simplex virus lesions in the vagina are an indication for caesarean section.
- Ophthalmia neonatorum is due to chlamydia (66%) or gonorrhoea (33%). However, a neonate with sticky eyes is more likely to have staphylococcal conjunctivitis or a blocked tear duct.

Post-natally acquired infections carried by nurses, doctors and parents.
- Staphyloccocal conjunctivitis or skin infections (umbilicus).
- Oral and perineal candida.

Differential diagnosis of neonatal fever.
- Infection.
- Dehydration fever.
- Heart failure.
- Intracranial haemorrhage.
Investigation of fever. As for convulsions.

SEIZURES
= repetitive, jerky movements.

Incidence. 4/1000 live births.
Clinically. Jerks, twitches, apnoea, alterations in tone, impaired level of consciousness.
Differential diagnosis of neonatal seizures
* Normal jerks on awakening, agitation of a hungry baby, Moro, jitteriness.
* Tetany.
* Tetanus (not in Britain).

Aetiology.	Day 0-3	4-7
• 5% Developmental anomalies (CNS, heart)	++	+
• 50% Perinatal complications (trauma, anoxia, intracranial haemorrhage, cerebral oedema)	+	
• Infection (bacterial or viral meningitis)		+
• Hypoglycaemia	+	
• Hypocalcaemia	+	++
• Jaundice		+

Occasionally: hyponatraemia, hypomagnesaemia, organic acidosis.
Investigation. Blood glucose, calcium, magnesium, bilirubin, sodium. Blood gases. Ultrasound scan of head. CSF for microscopy and culture. Blood for culture and viral titres. Culture swabs from nose, throat, and umbilicus. CxR. Urine culture. Urine for abnormal amino acids or reducing sugars.
Treatment. Protect the airway. Diazepam > paraldehyde for epileptic status. Phenytoin > phenobarbitone for frequent fits. Treat the cause.
Prognosis. The later the onset of seizures the better the prognosis. Simple hypocalcaemia and subarachnoid haemorrhage have an excellent prognosis.

HYPOGLYCAEMIA
= glucose <2.5 mmol/l.
Aetiology. Commoner in small for gestational age (SGA) babies than premature babies. Occasionally due to liver failure or an inborn error of metabolism.
Clinically. Jittery, episodes of apnoea, convulsions.
Management. Prevent hypoglycaemia by giving frequent feeds to neonates at risk. Treat hypoglycaemia with oral feeds or i.v. dextrose.

HYPOCALCAEMIA
= plasma calcium < 1.8 mmol/l.
Incidence. Uncommon. Due to:
* Early hypocalcaemia (day 1-3 after delivery) in any very sick baby.
* Late hypocalcaemia (day 4-7) used to occur in neonates given phosphate-rich cows' milk before parathyroid function had fully developed.

Clinically. Hypocalcaemia in a neonate causes jitteriness, tetany, seizures.
Treatment. Calcium gluconate i.v. or orally.
Prognosis. Late hypocalcaemia has a good prognosis.

ANAEMIA
Aetiology.
- Haemolytic disease of the newborn.
- Haemorrhage or haematoma.
- Genetic abnormality of red cells or haemoglobin.
- Premature neonates may develop a dilutional anaemia due to relatively rapid growth compared to erythropoiesis.
- Transfusion between twins sharing one placenta so that one twin is polycythaemic and the other is anaemic.

Clinically. Pale, tachycardia, tachypnoea, hepatomegaly (heart failure).
Investigation and treatment. See 'Haematology'.

NEONATAL JAUNDICE
Incidence. 30-50% of neonates are jaundiced during the first week.
Pathophysiology. If more than about 340 micromoles/litre of unconjugated bilirubin accumulates in the neonate it precipitates in the basal ganglia causing kernicterus. The bilirubin level at which kernicterus occurs is reduced by anoxia, hypoglycaemia, acidosis, hypothermia, prematurity and reduced protein binding of bilirubin.
Aetiology. Usually 'physiological jaundice'.
1. Hepatic enzyme defect
   - Physiological jaundice and prolonged physiological jaundice
   - Gilbert's (common but mild), Galactosaemia (rare but severe)
2. Increased haemolysis
   - Maternal antibodies (haemolytic disease of the newborn)
   - Red cell defect (spherocytosis, G6PDH deficiency, thalassaemia)
   - Resolving haematoma
   - Polycythaemia
   - Infection (septicaemia, UTI, 'TORCH')
   - Drugs
3. Hepatitis
4. Biliary obstruction
5. Reduced protein binding of bilirubin (low albumin, sulphonamides).
Clinically. The jaundiced neonate sometimes develops kernicterus - becomes lethargic, twitchy, hypertonic and feeds poorly. Convulsions and respiratory failure follow. Up to 2/3 die and the remainder have cerebral palsy.

21

Investigation. See chapter on 'Liver disease'.
Jaundice on day 1 - test for haemolytic disease (see below).
Jaundice after 4 days - screen for infection, see 'hepatitis'.
Treatment. See below under 'rhesus haemolytic disease'.

Physiological jaundice
Incidence. Occurs in 30-50% of neonates.
Aetiology. Occurs 2-7 days after delivery, when normal haemolysis of fetal haemoglobin overloads the hepatic glucoronyl transferase (GT) available. The serum contains increased unconjugated bilirubin but the urine and stools are normal coloured. If GT activity increases more slowly than usual physiological jaundice is prolonged. Caused by: prematurity, birth anoxia, hypothyroidism, fluid deprivation, breast milk jaundice.

Rhesus haemolytic disease of the newborn
Incidence. Less than 1% of pregnancies (seldom affects the first).
Pathology. Rhesus (Rh) antibody (Ab) made by a Rh-negative mother, crosses the placenta and haemolyses fetal blood in a Rh-positive fetus.
Clinical syndromes
- Hydrops fetalis = severe anaemia (cardiac failure, usually stillborn).
- Jaundice = unconjugated bilirubin accumulates as soon as the placenta separates and is evident within a few hours of delivery, kernicterus can develop rapidly. Variable anaemia and heart failure.
- Gradual anaemia (erythroblastosis fetalis). Mild jaundice, progressive anaemia, heart failure and hepatosplenomegaly.

Prevent sensitization.
- Do not transfuse a woman with incompatible blood.
- Give anti-D if a Rh-negative woman has vaginal bleeding in pregnancy, and within 48 hours of childbirth to destroy any fetal red cells that have entered the maternal circulation.
- Once sensitization has occurred plasma exchange transfusion and plasmapheresis might reduce Ab levels and allow a live birth.

Antenatal care.
- Ab titres on Rh-negative women in the first trimester, repeated at 28, 34 and 38 weeks. If Abs are found, repeat frequently to assess the need for amniocentesis to measure bilirubin and Ab levels in the liquor.
- Intrauterine transfusion can be used to maintain an affected fetus until early delivery at 32 weeks gestation.
- Phenobarbitone given to the mother for 2 weeks prior to delivery induces GT activity and increases neonatal bilirubin conjugation.

Post-natal. Cord blood for Rhesus and ABO grouping, haemoglobin, Coombs test and bilirubin. Reduce bilirubin level by:
- Phototherapy and a high fluid intake.
- Exchange transfusion.
- Salt-free human albumin infusion (protein binding of bilirubin).
- Phenobarbitone induces fetal GT but is seldom used.

Prognosis. 95% of those born alive will survive.

ABO haemolytic disease of the newborn

Anti-A or Anti-B haemolysins are generated by a group O mother and cause mild disease in a fetus with blood group A or B. This occurs in 0.5% of pregnancies (as likely to affect the firstborn as subsequent pregnancies).

Neonatal hepatitis
Aetiology.
- Congenital hepatic infection ('TORCH')
- Any severe infection (UTI, septicaemia)
- Drugs
- Alpha-1-antitrypsin deficiency

Clinically. Obstructive jaundice. See chapter on 'Liver disease'.
Prognosis. 33% die as neonates, 33% develop cirrhosis, 33% recover.

VOMITING, DIARRHOEA, CONSTIPATION, OBSTRUCTION
See 'Gastrointestinal Tract'.

Necrotising enterocolitis
Incidence. 1-5% of babies admitted to a neonatal unit. Affects 10% of babies weighing less than 1500 grams at birth. Other risk factors: umbilical catheter, sepsis, shock, cows' milk feeding.
Pathology. Ischaemic necrosis of bowel.
Clinically. Intestinal obstruction (vomiting and distension).
Investigation. Abdominal X-ray shows gas in the wall of distended bowel.
Treatment. Nil by mouth, aspirate stomach, give i.v. fluids and antibiotics. Resect necrotic bowel if there is no improvement after 24 hours.
Prognosis. 40% mortality. Survivors often develop an intestinal stricture.

CONGENITAL MALFORMATIONS
See the relevant system.

6. CHILD HEALTH

PREVENTION
- **Primary prevention** is the prevention of disease. Encouraging healthy behaviour by legislation (seat belts), advertising ("smoking can damage your unborn baby"), health education for parents and children (the "Green Cross Code"), opportunistic education ("Do you have a gate guard for the stairs?"), and social support. Immunisations, and genetic counselling.
- **Secondary prevention** is the detection of asymptomatic abnormalities (disease and developmental defects) by screening, e.g. Guthrie test, and developmental screening. Parents are often right if they suspect that their child is abnormal but they may not identify the abnormality correctly and often miss abnormalities. For example, 85% of the parents of children with amblyopia are unaware that their child has a visual problem.
- **Tertiary prevention** is the limitation of disease and disability by the early detection and provision of care for symptomatic abnormalities.

SCREENING
Screening = The presumptive identification of unrecognised disease or defect by application of examinations and tests which can be applied rapidly. Screening tests are not diagnostic - they merely identify those, apparently well, children who are more likely to have disease or dysfunction.

A condition is suitable for screening if:
- It is **important**.
- There is an **early asymptomatic stage**.
- The **natural history of the disorder is understood**.
- An appropriate screening **test is available**.
- An acceptable and **effective treatment** is available.
- The **indications for treatment are agreed**.
- The **cost of screening should be reasonable** in comparison to other uses of limited resources.

A screening test is appropriate if it is:
- **Acceptable** (not painful).
- **Repeatable**.
- **Sensitive** (is almost always positive when the disease is present).
- **Specific** (is almost always negative when the disease is not present).
- **Simple**, quick and easy to interpret.

Developmental screening
A set of procedures carried out on all 'normal' children to identify those who **may** have undetected abnormalities.

Child health surveillance
Oversight of the physical, intellectual, social and emotional, health and development of children. Includes developmental assessment.

Under regulations introduced on 1st April 1990, GPs with appropriate training and experience will be paid a fee for each child under the age of 5 years for whom they have agreed to provide a child health surveillance service. This service is also provided in District Health Authority Clinics by Clinical Medical Officers.

Developmental assessment
A set of procedures (questions, observations, examinations and tests) designed to **establish** the stage of development and deviations from normal. Developmental assessment covers:
- Gross motor (sitting, standing, walking, running).
- Fine motor (grasp, fine manipulation).
- Language (hearing, speech, understanding).
- Social development (smiling, response to strangers).

Many parents have inaccurate memories of their childrens' development, but inviting comparisons with other children of the same age and sex (girls develop faster) can assist recall.

You are not safe to carry out developmental screening until you:
- Can use centile charts, including decimal age and corrections for mid-parental height.
- Can use vision and hearing tests appropriate to children of all ages.
- Are aware of the range of normal for each developmental milestone. The best way to learn the acceptable and unacceptable variations in child development is to carry out assessments on lots of children.

SURVEILLANCE PROGRAMME
The following timetable for developmental assessments does not cover children with suspected abnormalities who should be referred or assessed more frequently. Children who move to the area need immediate review because the children of mobile families are under particular stresses and often evade preventive care.

Neonate
See chapter on 'The Neonate'.

Late 'neonatal' (3 to 6 weeks old).
- History of feeding problems, maternal depression.
- Repeat neonatal examination: vision (no squint, follows face through 180°), hearing (turns to sound through 180°). Demonstrate to mother that her baby sees, hears and responds by smiling.
- Advice about feeding, clothing.

Infant (7 to 8 months).
- Gross motor. Speech. Vision: Stycar rolling ball test.
- Hearing: turns to sounds such as Nuffield Rattle or "MEG Warbler".
- Social: separation and stranger anxiety develop around 8 months so do the assessment before then if possible.
- Congenital abnormalities: undescended testes, hips.
- Health education: diet, accident prevention, language stimulation, explanation of separation anxiety.

12 to 15 months
- Examination mainly to reassure parents but congenital dislocation of hips and spastic paraplegia can present with delayed walking. Vision: cover test for squint, test vision with rolling balls. Test hearing by distraction (after 13 months children are too restless to do this).
- Advice on: diet, accident prevention, language stimulation, coping with separation anxiety.

18 months
- Language and play (often carried out by health visitors).
- Blood for haemoglobin if at risk of anaemia (food fads, vegetarian).
- Advice on: language and play stimulation, behaviour problems such as sleep disturbance and tantrums.

24 to 30 months (optional)
- Gait, fine motor function, speech and language, vision, mental development, testes, height and weight (measure parents' height before diagnosing growth failure).
- Language and play stimulation (the parents often say 'I never knew he could do that' when they see their child cooperating with the developmental testing). Consider playgroup.

3.5 to 4.5 years (pre-school)
- Vision test by orthoptist if possible (squint and amblyopia). Hearing test.

- Full physical examination. Assess all aspects of development with particular attention to socialisation skills.
- Advice on: playgroup or nursery school can help prepare mother and child for the separation on starting 'proper school'.

SUMMARY OF KEY DEVELOPMENTAL MILESTONES
A 6 week old child would usually:
- Hold head transiently horizontal if held in ventral suspension.
- Smile back at mother.
- Retain some primitive reflexes such as the Moro response.
- Turn through 180° to seek mother's voice if held sitting upright.

A 7 month old child would usually:
- Sit without support (75%), stand with support (93%).
- Bear his weight on his hands when prone (60%).
- Transfer a 1 inch brick from hand to hand (63%).
- Utter 2 syllable babble ('mama').

A 12 month old child would usually:
- Walk with one hand held.
- Release bricks into the examiner's hand (60%).
- Say 3 words with meaning (75%).

A child of 30 months would usually:
- Kick a ball accurately (75%), throw a ball with one hand (80%).
- Make a tower of 8 cubes.
- Say 4 word sentences (80%).
- Be dry by day (90% of girls, 70% of boys).

A child of 54 months (4.5 years) would usually:
- Hop on one leg (65%). Build a 6 brick pyramid (60%).
- Dress themselves (70% of girls, 60% of boys).
- Hold a clear conversation (76%).
- Be dry at night (85% of girls, 80% of boys).

HANDICAP
A disability is a loss or reduction of functional capacity. A handicap is the disadvantage or restriction of activity caused by a disability. A concise review of the management of handicap is given in chapter 40 of 'Child Care in General Practice', which is listed in the bibliography.

7. EDUCATION

LEGISLATION
Education Act 1944
Every child over 5 years old and under the school leaving age must receive full time education. The school leaving age is the end of the spring or summer term next following the child's 16th birthday. If the child does not attend school, and the parents are unable to prove that the child is receiving an adequate education at home, the parents can be prosecuted. The Local Education Authority (LEA) must provide medical and dental treatment for pupils. Physical examinations are usually carried out at age 5, 11 and 16. Abnormalities are found in 2 to 20% of 5 year olds, but most of these have been identified by parents, child surveillance clinics, health visitors or teachers.

The Education Act 1981
This developed from the recommendation of the Warnock Report 1978 that 'All children should have education appropriate to their needs'.
* Under age 5 District Health Authorities (DHAs) are required to identify children who may have special educational needs. The DHA must inform the parents that their child may have special needs, inform the parents of relevant voluntary organisations and designate a doctor from whom the parents can seek further advice. The DHA must inform the LEA and refer the child to a district handicap team (Child Development Team). After age 2 a full 'statement of special educational needs' (SSEN) is required.
* Over age 5 the LEA is responsible for identifying children with special educational needs. The LEA must inform the parents, nursing officer, social services, and DHA. The DHA will appoint a doctor to assess the child. The designated doctor may involve other professionals. After the assessment a SSEN is presented to the parents. If the parents disagree with the SSEN they can appeal to the DHA, a local appeal committee or the Secretary of State for Health.
* SSEN must be reviewed every 12 months Between the age of 12.5 and 14.5 years a full reassessment is required unless the SSEN has been revoked earlier.
* The LEA is responsible for providing a range of special educational services, special education officers, needs advisors and support staff. LEA psychologists coordinate multi-professional assessments.

Education Act 1988
National curriculum with 'testing' at 7, 11, 14 and 16 years. Children with a SSEN can be allowed to omit part or all of the national curriculum.

EDUCATIONAL PROBLEMS
Incidence. About 20% of children have special educational needs. Most attend normal schools, but children with more severe difficulties (2%) attend special schools. Of those attending special schools most have general learning difficulties, many have physical handicaps including blindness and deafness, some are emotionally disturbed.

Classification.
- General intellectual limitation as measured by IQ testing.
- Specific learning difficulties such as dyslexia.
- Physical handicap.
- Persistent or recurrent illness.
- Neurotic illness including school refusal.
- Psychotic disorders.
- Conduct disorders including truancy.
- Parents who prevent their children from attending school or studying at home.

SCHOOL ABSENCE
Differential diagnosis of school absence.
- **Illness.** This accounts for 90% of school absence.
- **Truancy.** Adolescent boys with poor academic records who decide, usually without their parents' knowledge, not to attend school. Often from large disorganised families from social classes IV and V. May be involved in anti-social behaviour.
- **Parental refusal**: the child may be required to work in or outside the home, the parent may need the child's company.
- **School refusal.** Affects prepubertal children. Girls slightly more often than boys. Often an only child. Normal intelligence. Shy, quiet and hard working. Parents are indulgent and predominantly from social classes I, II and III. The father is often a remote figure.
- **Separation anxiety.** A young child may worry that his mother will be hurt if he leaves her.
- **School phobia.** A young child who has been bullied by other children or frightened by a teacher suddenly develops an irrational fear of school. Often presents somatic symptoms in order to remain at home.
- **Social phobia.**

Management of school absence.
- Each school should have policies for certifying and responding to different frequencies of school absence.

- Try to modify circumstances at school or at home which are causing the school absence.
- Treat psychiatric or physical illness in the child.
- Set a day to return to school in consultation with the child and his parents. Consider arranging a graded return starting with part-time attendance.
- Truancy can sometimes be controlled only by admission to a boarding school or residential home.

SPEECH DELAY
Normal speech development
Normal speech depends on:

- Hearing others speaking.
- Understanding the meaning of words.
- Understanding the relationship between words and the meaning of phrases.
- Putting words together in a meaningful way.
- Making the correct sounds.

Normal speech development starts with babbling at age 6 months. The meaningful use of words starts at 12 months, and the vocabulary includes 50 words by 18 months old. Sentences appear at age 2 years, and most children can engage an adult in conversation by age 5.

Abnormal speech development
Incidence. At school entry 5% of children are unintelligible through poor articulation, 1% have a limited vocabulary and 0.1% have severe language difficulty that is not due to deafness or mental retardation.

Aetiology.
- Deaf (usually due to glue ear).
- Idiopathic (often familial).
- Specific language disorder.
- Global mental retardation.
- Specific brain damage.
- Dysarthria = poor articulation due to defects of mouth and tongue: cleft palate, cerebral palsy, cranial nerve palsies.
- Dysphonia = disorders of the vocal cords.
- Dysrhythmia = disorder of breathing control.
- Psychiatric: autism, elective mutism.

Management. Refer for assessment by a speech therapist.
- Idiopathic articulation defects usually resolve spontaneously. A little extra time spent talking with the parents each day can hasten the process. Increased incidence of specific learning defects (dyslexia, dysgraphia).

- Impaired comprehension should be regarded as a form of mental retardation. Refer for a full assessment of educational needs.
- The management of deafness is covered in the Ear, nose and throat chapter.

LEARNING DIFFICULTIES
Normal learning
Normal reading, writing, drawing and counting depends on;
- Seeing symbols (although the sensations of fine position sense and touch can compensate).
- Understanding the meaning of symbols.
- Understanding the relationship between symbols and the meaning of patterns.
- Putting symbols together in a meaningful way.
- Making symbols that are comprehensible to others.

Most 3 year olds can copy a circle and a cross and rudimentary drawings of 'mummy' follow. In the British school system reading and copying letters is introduced at age 5.

Learning difficulties
Incidence. 10% of children. Boys (2:1). Commoner in social class V.
Differential diagnosis of learning difficulties.
- Specific learning defects (commonest learning difficulty).
- Inadequate teaching at home or at school.
- Frequent school absences.
- Poor concentration may be due to emotional disturbance, lack of motivation to learn, the effects of medication or drugs, and epilepsy.
- Mental retardation.
- Sensory defects (poor vision or deafness).
- Motor defects (ataxia, weakness).

Management. Refer for a full assessment of educational needs.

Specific learning defects
Often familial. Males from social classes IV and V, without a dominant side are at risk. Associated with clumsiness, speech delay, and behaviour problems.
- **Dyslexia** = difficulty learning to read. Idiopathic or associated with lesions in the dominant hemisphere.
- **Dysgraphia** = difficulty writing. The writing may be correct but poorly formed (motor problem), irregular and frequently wrong (ataxic), or full of spelling mistakes.
- **Dyscalculia** = difficulty with simple arithmetic.

8. PSYCHIATRY

BEHAVIOUR PROBLEMS

Assessment
- Ask the parents to describe the problem with actual examples. Be aware of the emotional content of their description. Do the parents blame a particular event or person for the problem?
- Ask the child for his version of the problem. Arrange a separate appointment (do not send the parents out of the room).
- Verify the details with other sources: teachers, social workers.
- Consider the problem within the context of the child's age, physical abilities and social circumstances. Bed-wetting is normal in infants. Deafness may present as 'not doing as he is told'.
- Consider the family dynamics. Who has got the real problem? Are the parents' expectations inappropriate or are their perceptions distorted?
- Consider who or what is the target of the behaviour problem. Misbehaviour that is 'strange' or without a target is more likely to be due to an organic disorder.

Management
- What do the parents expect you to do and achieve? Some families wish a scapegoated child to be removed into care and will generate crisis after crisis until they succeed.
- What are the parents willing to do to help their child? Behavioural problems can only improve if parents change their reactions towards the child. The parents' new behaviour must be consistent and provide clear limits to the child's behaviour.
- The parents need to be helped to develop a management plan. A 'cure' provided by the counsellor seldom works as well as one chosen by the parents.
- The counsellor can help the parents set achievable targets and analyse the reasons for success or failure. The parents will need encouragement because the child will use sulks, tantrums and tears to fight his parents' attempt to change his behaviour.
- The essence of behaviour therapy is to avoid rewarding unwanted behaviour (withdrawal of attention and privileges) and reward good behaviour (attention, small presents, star charts).

Sleep disturbance
Incidence. 10% of pre-school children are considered to be poor sleepers by their parents.

Aetiology.
- Trained to stay awake.
- Separation anxiety.
- Depression.
- Nightmares. Common. Age 8-10. Wakes terrified and remembering the dream.
- Night terrors. Age 4-7. Rare. The child half-wakes terrified and still dreaming. He cannot remember his dream when he wakes in the morning.
- Sleep walking. Very rare. Age 11-14. Walks half-awake and calm. No memory of the event on waking in the morning.
- Illness.

Management.
The majority of children with unacceptable sleep patterns have been "trained to stay awake". If a child is rewarded with a drink, a cuddle and a story if he wakes in the middle of the night, he will wake every night. If he is taken into his parents' bed when he cries, you can hardly blame him if he cries as soon as he is put into his cot. The child can be trained to sleep by:
- Responding to crying by attending to the child, but limiting the attention to excluding physical problems such as a sodden nappy.
- Not attending to the child as soon as he wakes, but waiting until he cries. Children often wake transiently at night.
- Gradually increasing the time the child is left to cry before attending.
- Not providing drinks, cuddles and stories.
- Sedatives are a last resort because they are often ineffective and sometimes make children hyperactive. If sedatives are given the parents should take the opportunity to modify their own pattern behaviour so as to encourage good sleeping habits when the sedative is withdrawn.

If one or both parents refuses to adhere to the regime one should consider whether they find some secondary gain in the child's behaviour. A woman who wishes to avoid intercourse may need a sleepless child as a chaperone.

Temper tantrums

Incidence. Commonest at age 5 years when 10% have at least 1 tantrum per week. Boys>girls. Single mother or ineffectual father are common circumstances.

Psychopathology. Tantrums represent an uncontrolled response to a frustrating situation. The behaviour becomes established if the child learns that his parents will give in to his demands if he has a tantrum.

Clinically. The child rampages around your consulting room ignoring the pitiful pleas of his parents.

Management. The parents should sit or stand near the child but say or do nothing until the tantrum is finished. He may be placed in a room without toys until he calms down ('time-out'). The child may need to be gently restrained from causing harm to himself, objects or people around him. He should not be bribed to stop, and imminent treats should be postponed so that the child does not interpret them as rewards for tantrums.

Prognosis. Many adults have tantrums. During tantrums toddlers may have blue breath holding attacks (see 'fits'), and older children may hyperventilate.

Hyperactive children

Incidence. Common. Boys>girls. The majority are otherwise normal but some show signs of minimal brain dysfunction syndrome. A few are mentally retarded or taking sedative drugs.

Clinically. 'Hyperactive' children do not move more than 'normal' children. However, their activity is disorganised, unrelated to generally accepted patterns of children's behaviour and devoid of consideration for others. They 'just won't stay still' or 'do as they are told'. As a consequence of this behaviour the children are often rejected by their parents, siblings and peers. They are prone to accidents and have learning problems.

Management. Reassure the parents that the child will improve with age. Stimulants such as methylphenidate can paradoxically inhibit hyperactivity. Occasional children benefit from an additive free diet. Behavioural therapy.

Prognosis. Hyperactivity persists into adolescence and adults remain impulsive and accident prone. A low IQ or conduct disorders are associated with a worse prognosis.

Conduct disorders

5% of 4 to12 year olds are noticeably aggressive and/or caught stealing. One third continue to be maladjusted in adolescence (vandalism, assault, promiscuity, rape, and truancy). Boys > girls.

Aetiology.

Usually primary:

- Unloved by parents or institutional carers.
- No consistent social training: disrupted family life.
- Trained to behave anti-socially. A child from a criminal family is not taught the concept of right and wrong. He may be taught that violence is the best method of getting what he wants. He has no compassion for those he hurts.
- A delinquent peer group.

Occasionally secondary:
- Neurosis, psychosis.
- Temporal lobe epilepsy, mental retardation, drug abuse.

Management. Drug therapy, behaviour therapy and psychoanalysis are of little or no benefit if the family is disorganised. Social work is of variable benefit. Local authority care may be needed.

Prognosis. Severe cases usually become worse in adult life. Early and repeated parenthood provides the next generation of maladjusted citizens (the 'cycle of deprivation').

Stealing

Many children occasionally steal small items. Frequent or large thefts may be:
- Comforting: thefts from parents in lieu of love.
- Proving: thefts of status objects carried out alone then displayed.
- Marauding: a group of children go out with the intention of stealing if the opportunity arises.
- Planned: a group of children steal a previously identified item.
- Thefts of food when hungry.
- Theft under the direction of parents.
- Theft of items needed by a sick parent.

EMOTIONAL DISORDERS
Affect 5% of pre-adolescent children and 2.5% of adolescent children.

Anxiety

Incidence. Common.
- Separation anxiety is a normal developmental stage (7 months). If prolonged or severe it causes emotional distress to both child and parents.
- Natural reaction to stresses (parental discord, neglect or abuse, change of home or school, bereavement).

Clinically.
- Simple separation anxiety and excessive fear of strangers (shy).
- Sleep disturbance. 'He won't lie down in his bed, he just screams'.
- School refusal (see 'Education' chapter).
- Physical symptoms: recurrent abdominal pains and headaches.
- Phobias and obsessions are uncommon but 3/4 persist into adult life.

Management. Allow older children to discuss their anxiety. Stresses should be modified if possible. Behavioural therapy or goal-orientated psychotherapy for obsessions and phobias.

Depression

Sadness is common in childhood. If depression is defined as prolonged sadness out of proportion to the child's situation, about 0.1% of 10 year olds and 1% of 15 year olds are depressed. Anti-depressant medication is as effective for children as for adults.

HABIT DISORDERS
- Nail-biting may reflect anxiety.
- Tics (see 'Neurology').
- Masturbation. A normal phase of development in young children. Persistent masturbation may reflect anxiety or boredom.

DISORDERS OF ELIMINATION

Enuresis

= involuntary voiding of urine at an age when control of micturition is normal.

Incidence. The average child is dry by day at age 2 and dry by night at age 3. Bed-wetting (nocturnal enuresis) is commoner in boys – 15% of 5 year olds and 5% of 10 year olds still wet their beds. Daytime enuresis (diurnal enuresis) is less common, commoner in girls, and is usually limited to a slight leak.

Aetiology.
- **Primary enuresis:** isolated developmental delay (often familial) > global developmental delay > anatomical abnormality (ectopic ureter), neuropathic bladder.
- **Secondary enuresis:** any illness or emotional upset, urinary tract infection. Occasionally polyuria (diabetes mellitus) or nocturnal epilepsy.

Management.
- **Nocturnal enuresis.** Urine culture. If urine is sterile consider: last drink at 6 pm, void before going to bed, alarm in the child's room set for 11 pm and 3 am. If this regime fails try an enuresis alarm or imipramine. Star charts are useful to document success but being dry is sufficient reward for most children.
- **Diurnal enuresis.** Urine culture and IVP. If normal teach pelvic floor exercises and a programme of gradually increasing the intervals between micturition.

Prognosis. Seldom persists beyond childhood.

Faecal soiling

Between the age of 1 and 3 most children come to be aware of the need to defaecate and learn to control the urge until they can reach a potty or toilet.

Incidence. 2% of boys and 1% of girls soil more than once each month at the age of 8. Half of these children had always soiled.

Aetiology.

- Delayed maturation of bowel control.
- Chronic constipation with overflow diarrhoea is common. May be due to a wilful avoidance of defaecation in a parent-child power struggle, a low fibre diet or medication. Rarely due to anatomical abnormality of the bowel.
- Encopresis = deliberate defaecation in inappropriate places. A symptom of grossly disturbed training or emotional upset.
- Faecal incontinence due to neurological or anatomical abnormality (meningomyelocele).
- Mental retardation.
- Diarrhoea.

Management. Treat constipation and diarrhoea if present. Family therapy combined with behaviour therapy often cures the problem for a while. Spontaneous cure by age 20 is invariable unless there is an anatomical abnormality.

EATING DISORDERS

Always plot the weight on a centile chart. Normal growth virtually excludes a serious problem.

Food refusal

20% of pre-adolescent children use food refusal as a means of gaining attention. It should be treated in the same way as food fads.

Food fads

Food fads are an extreme expression of the food preferences we all have. If parents permit their child to eat only what he wants they have only themselves to blame. Retraining involves giving the child the opportunity to eat the same food as the rest of the family with no alternatives. There should be no encouragement to eat. Food should not be provided except at mealtimes. The child will eat once he is hungry.

Anorexia nervosa and bulaemia

Affects 0.3% of adolescent girls (97% of cases). Tends to occur in families with a tendency to obesity or anorexia nervosa (not genetic). Social classes I and II. May start as conventional dieting but becomes a means of avoiding the sexual tensions of adolescence. The girl wishes to be lighter than is healthy.

She avoids food and will attempt to vomit any food she has been forced to eat. She becomes withdrawn but continues to work hard at school. As starvation develops she becomes hypothermic and asexual (amenorrhoea, breast atrophy). Some develop a pattern of bingeing and vomiting (bulaemia). 60% recover, 30% remain anorexic throughout adult life, 10% die from starvation and suicide.

Obesity

An abnormally high percentage of body fat. This is best measured by skin-fold thickness. Weight may reflect increased muscle mass.

Differential diagnosis.

1. Usually overeating: calorie intake regularly exceeds metabolic requirements. Girls>boys. The mother is often obese. Rural. Social class IV and V.
   - High calorie intake. Initially the parents offer the child too much food but overeating becomes a habit for the child.
   - Low metabolic needs: constitutional or due to inactivity.
2. Endocrine abnormalities: hypothyroidism, Cushing's syndrome (steroid therapy), polycystic ovaries, Klinefelter's syndrome.
3. Hypothalamic lesion.

Complications. Social. Menstrual (early menarche, irregular menses). Medical (increased mortality, diabetes, hypertension).

Treatment. Diet. Activity. Self-help groups. Appetite suppressants and surgery are rarely indicated.

DRUG ABUSE

Many children experiment with a variety of drugs, but alcohol and cigarettes are the only common addictions. More boys become regular abusers. As the child becomes addicted parents often notice behaviour changes with withdrawal, stealing, and temper outbursts. School performance declines. Parents may be horrified by finding evidence of drug abuse but some consider alcohol and cigarettes to be part of growing up. If the parent-child relationship has broken down a referral to child guidance and local self-help groups may be appropriate. If the child is forced to leave home he will inevitably enter the criminal culture associated with drug abuse. Once physical dependence has developed withdrawal is characterized by anxiety, tremor, sweating, tachycardia, nausea, insomnia. Withdrawal may need to monitored in hospital. Excepting tobacco and alcohol the common drugs of abuse are:

- Marihuana (cannabis) is smoked for its euphoric effect. Typically it is used intermittently with little effect on social functioning.

- Solvents, usually toluene vapour from glue, are inhaled from bags for their euphoric effect. Adolescent males from disturbed families become users through peer group pressures. Physical addiction does not occur. Acute intoxication can lead to confusion, hallucinations, vomiting, convulsions, collapse. Renal or hepatic impairment is usually mild and transient. Ten deaths per year (asphyxiated by the bag holding the glue, falls or inhalation of vomit).
- Stimulants (amphetamines and related drugs, cocaine) are used in 'acid house' parties for their euphoric effect.
- Hallucinogenics.
- Sedatives.
- Narcotics. Heroin can be heated and inhaled or injected (risk of Hepatitis B and AIDS). Look for needle marks, tender hepatomegaly and jaundice. Methadone liquid can be used to facilitate gradual withdrawal of narcotics or maintain a socially stable addict who does not wish to stop. Addicts with poor social circumstances benefit from the services of a drug dependency clinic.

PSYCHOSIS

The child's appreciation of his environment is distorted. This may present as withdrawal, impaired learning or the expression of frank delusions and hallucinations.

Incidence. Rare.

Aetiology.

1. Toxic confusional state.
   - Usually alcoholic. Occasionally other drugs of abuse.
   - Sometimes diabetic ketoacidosis or hypoglycaemia.
   - Febrile delirium is common but seldom severe.
   - Medication. Steroids, anticonvulsants.
   - Encephalitis.
2. Epilepsy.
3. Depression.
4. Schizophrenia (in adolescents).
5. Progressive cerebral damage (see 'CNS - Dementia').
6. Autism.

Differential diagnosis (mad, sad, bad, dull).

- Psychosis.
- Neurosis.
- Conduct disorder.
- Mental subnormality.

Autism

Impaired understanding of visual and auditory information.

Incidence. Occurs in 3/10,000 children. 75% boys. Develops before age 3. There is more concordance in identical twins than non-identical twins.

Clinically. The child is withdrawn (avoids eye contact), language development is absent (50%) or severely retarded (repetition of what he hears), dislikes any change in his routine and will play monotonously for hours. Manipulative skills are preserved. Most are intellectually retarded but there may be islands of intact intellectual functioning.

Prognosis. Social language and self care can be taught by repetition. Two-thirds require institutional care. One third develop epilepsy. Autism does not develop into adult schizophrenia.

9. GENETIC ABNORMALITIES

SIGNIFICANCE
Genetic abnormalities are found in 3% of livebirths and 10% of stillbirths. About 5% of children admitted to hospital have a genetic disorder and such disorders cause 10% of childhood deaths in hospital.

PREVENTION
Genetic defects cannot be cured but the incidence of handicap can be reduced by:
- Laws and taboos against consanguineous relationships. 3% of children born to parents who are cousins are homozygous for autosomal recessive conditions. This rises to 10% for incestuous relationships.
- Genetic counselling and contraception.
- Antenatal screening with selective abortion.

The degree of handicap can be limited by:
- Neonatal screening with early treatment.
- Special educational provision and good medical care for affected children.
- Social support for affected families.

Genetic counselling
- Define the genetic abnormality, if any, affecting the index case. This requires a detailed physical examination and laboratory investigations including chromosome analysis.
- Determine whether a genetic abnormality is a new mutation or inherited. As many relatives as possible should be examined, and a family tree should be constructed. Laboratory investigations may detect sub-clinical abnormalities in relatives of an index case.
- Inform the parents of the diagnosis, proposed management and prognosis for the affected child. Discuss the risk of subsequent children being affected.
- An affected child should be given the opportunity to discuss the same information once they are able to understand the diagnosis.
- Relatives may also need counselling.
- Allow the parents to discuss feelings of guilt, anxiety, anger and sadness.
- Couples at risk of producing an affected child may choose contraception, sterilisation, pregnancy with antenatal screening, artificial insemination by donor (if the man has an autosomal dominant condition), or treatment to reduce the risk of recurrence of a polygenic abnormality.
- Obstetricians and paediatricians should be warned of the risk of recurrence when a carrier or a couple with an affected child conceive.

Antenatal screening

- Maternal blood for alpha-fetoprotein (AFP) in the first trimester.
- Chorionic villous sampling through the cervix at 8 weeks of gestation. Placental tissue can be cultured to determine the karyotype and identify defective enzymes or haemoglobin. 5% miscarriage rate.
- Amniocentesis at 16 weeks gestation. A raised AFP suggests an open neural tube defect. Fetal skin cells in the amniotic fluid are sent for karyotyping to determine sex and identify abnormal karyotypes such as Trisomy 21. Culture fetal cells to detect enzyme defects. 1% miscarriage rate.
- Ultrasound at 19 weeks gestation for neural tube defects.
- Fetoscopy at 15 to 20 weeks has been largely replaced by ultrasound. Useful for fetal blood sampling. 5% miscarriage rate.

CHROMOSOMAL ABNORMALITIES

4/1,000 live births have a chromosomal abnormality. About 5% of these are inherited, the remainder arise during formation of the gametes, or in the early embryo. In general, the risk of recurrence is 1–5% unless one of the parents is carrying the abnormal chromosome.

Abnormal numbers of autosomes

These are associated with low birth weight, failure to thrive, hypotonia, developmental delay and an odd appearance (Trisomy 21 = Down's syndrome).

Structural abnormalities of autosomes

Those involving re-arrangement without deletion of genetic material are asymptomatic in 90% of cases. Deletion of part of an autosome often results in severe malformations. Complete absence of an autosome is invariably lethal in the first trimester.

Abnormal numbers of sex chromosomes

These are often asymptomatic until adolescence. Common features are the failure to develop secondary sexual characteristics, abnormal stature and fat distribution, and mental retardation. Turner's syndrome (45,XO), Klinefelter's syndrome (47,XXY), Superfemales (47,XXX), XYY syndrome.

SINGLE GENE DEFECTS

Occur in 1% of live births.

Autosomal recessive defects

Occur in 0.25% of live births. Both parents must carry the abnormal gene. On average 1/4 of the children of heterozygous parents will be affected. The defect is only clinically expressed in the homozygous state although sub-clinical abnormalities may be detectable in heterozygotes. Often an enzyme defect: phenylketonuria, homocystinuria, galactosaemia, storage diseases (Tay Sachs), cystic fibrosis. An autosomal recessive defect generally reduces the life expectancy more than an autosomal dominant defect.

Intermediate defects

These are expressed in a mild form in the heterozygote. Sickle cell trait is the heterozygous expression of the gene causing Sickle cell anaemia.

Autosomal dominant defects

Occur in 0.7% of live births. Half the children of an affected individual are affected. The gene is expressed to varying extents in heterozygotes so some appear to be normal. Some are expressed more frequently in one sex than the other. New mutations are frequent. Often complex syndromes: achondroplasia, Huntingdon's chorea, tuberous sclerosis, neurofibromatosis.

X-linked recessive defects

Usually affect males. Females have two X-chromosomes so they seldom express any defect although they carry the gene into the next generation. Haemophilia is the classical example.

Y-linked defects

These have not been recognised.

X-linked dominant defects

These are twice as common in females because they have twice as many X-chromosomes to go wrong. Vitamin D resistant rickets is one of the few examples.

POLYGENIC ABNORMALITIES

Occur in 2% of live births: anencephaly, spina bifida cystica, cleft lip, congenital heart disease, coeliac disease, insulin dependent diabetes, hare lip, congenital dislocation of the hip.

The predisposition to each of these abnormalities is transmitted by several genes which are not necessarily on the same chromosome. The expression of the abnormality depends on environmental factors. In general the risk of recurrence is 1 to 5% depending on the abnormality. The risk of recurrence is often greater if:

- The index case is severely affected.
- The index case is the 'wrong' sex for the condition. The incidence of pyloric stenosis recurring in subsequent children is 2% after an affected boy and 10% after an affected girl.
- Several first degree relatives are affected.

10. RESPIRATORY DISEASE

EPIDEMIOLOGY OF RESPIRATORY DISEASES
1. **Acute infections of the upper respiratory tract** affect the average child 4 times each year. A GP will diagnose 300 new episodes of coryza, pharyngitis and tonsillitis each year.
2. **Acute infections of the lower respiratory tract** affect 1 child in 10 each year. A GP will diagnose 75 cases of laryngotracheitis (croup), bronchitis, bronchiolitis, pneumonia, pertussis, and influenza each year.
3. **Chronic infections of the lower respiratory tract** affect less than one child on each GP's list. Bronchiectasis and tuberculosis are uncommon. Lung abscess is rare.
4. **Asthma** affects one child in 10.
5. **Congenital abnormalities** affect <1 child per GP.
6. **Neonatal problems** are discussed in another chapter.
7. **Others:** aspiration, neoplasia.

INFECTIONS OF THE UPPER RESPIRATORY TRACT

Common cold (coryza)
Aetiology. Viral infection of nasal passages by Rhinovirus, Respiratory Syncytial Virus (RSV), influenza, parainfluenza, adenovirus.
Clinically. Incubation 3 days. Main symptoms: nasal obstruction and discharge (mucoid or purulent). Associated symptoms: sneezing, headache, cough. Pre-school children commonly have fever, mild diarrhoea and vomiting. Babies feed poorly due to nasal obstruction. Illness lasts 7 to 14 days.
Differential diagnosis of nasal discharge.
* Prodromal symptoms of a specific infection: measles, diphtheria.
* Foreign body in nose (unilateral foul bloodstained discharge).
* Allergic rhinitis (persistent mucoid discharge, no fever).
* Sinusitis (facial pain) is rare before puberty.
Complications. Commonly: nosebleeds; secondary bacterial infection of nose, pharyngitis, otitis media. Sometimes: lower respiratory tract infection, sinusitis, febrile convulsions, cot death.
Management. Explain expected course of illness and acceptable symptoms. List warning signs such as tachypnoea, poor feeding, apathy. Diet and activity as tolerated. Encourage fluids. Prescribe:
* Paracetamol for fever and pain.
* Simple linctus (sugar free) if the parents 'must have something for the cough'.

45

- Normal saline nose drops as often as required for infants with feeding or sleeping problems. Ephedrine 0.5% nosedrops for resistant cases (rebound if used more than 5 days).
- Antibiotics if a complication has developed.

Pharyngitis and tonsillitis

Aetiology. 2/3 viral (adenovirus + viruses causing coryza), 1/3 Group A beta-haemolytic streptococcus.

Epidemiology. Affects more than one in ten children each year. Most common between 2 and 8 years old. Average GP consulted 200 times each year (half tonsillitis, half pharyngitis).

Clinically. Sudden onset of sore throat, fever and malaise. Often associated with coryza, cough, cervical adenopathy, anorexia, vomiting, abdominal pain, headache and meningism. Unilateral conjunctivitis suggests adenovirus. Pharyngitis is typified by a red pharynx but there may be ulcers and petechiae. Tonsillitis is diagnosed in the presence of enlarged, red tonsils ± exudate.

Complications.

1. Bacterial infections

- **Peritonsillar abscess (quinsy).** A GP will see 4 cases each year. Commonest in adolescence. Very sore throat, trismus, drooling, toxic, high fever, tonsillitis with swelling of adjacent pharynx, cervical swelling. Risk of airways obstruction. Need parenteral penicillin. Usually require admission. A few need surgical drainage.
- **Retropharyngeal abscess.** Rare. Toddler who is toxic and drooling. Stridor, prefers neck flexed. Posterior pharynx may bulge forwards, risk of airways obstruction. Admit to an ENT unit for lateral X-ray of pharynx, surgical drainage, and antibiotics.
- **Cervical abscess.** A GP sees 1 case every few years. Usually responds to antibiotics although some require surgical drainage. In atypical cases consider tuberculosis.
- **Chronic tonsillitis.** Common before puberty. Persistently red tonsils with malaise and recurrent acute tonsillitis. May respond to prolonged courses of penicillin. Check that there is no other organic disease (Urine culture, CxR, FBC, dental opinion). If the symptoms reported by the parents' are not supported by your examination, consider whether the parents have the problem (emotional or social). See 'Indications for tonsillectomy'.
- **Chronic adenoid hypertrophy.** See 'Ear, nose and throat'.

2. Complications of beta-haemolytic streptococcal infection.
   * Scarlet fever (see 'Infections').
   * Post-streptococcal glomerulonephritis (see 'Kidney and urinary tract').
   * Rheumatic fever and chorea (see 'Cardiovascular system').

Differential diagnosis of sore throat.
* Pharyngitis.
* Tonsillitis and its complications.
* Mouth ulcers.
* Foreign body such as impacted fish bone.
* Referred pain (teeth, ear, lymph nodes).
* Psychogenic.
* Agranulocytosis or leukaemia.

In the infant and toddler the differential diagnosis includes all the causes of fever (see infectious diseases).

Investigation.
In atypical cases consider throat swab for culture, full blood count, Paul Bunnell, urine culture, lateral X-ray of neck. When there is meningism the diagnosis may require lumbar puncture.

Treatment.
1. **Antibiotics**. Penicillin V > erythromycin. Avoid ampicillin or amoxycillin (cause a rash when given for glandular fever).

   Definite indications for antibiotics: severe illness, bacterial complications, previous rheumatic fever or nephritis (10 day course), exacerbation of chronic suppurative tonsillitis, reduced immunity or cystic fibrosis.

   Possible indication: bacterial epidemic in a residential school.

   Questionable indications:
   * To reassure the parents: antibiotics are expected by the majority of parents who have decided to take their child to the doctor. If you decide not to prescribe you must be prepared to spend time explaining why. Remember that for every 100,000 prescriptions for penicillin: 1 person will die from anaphylaxis, 100 will have a severe reaction and 10,000 will have a minor reaction such as a rash or gastrointestinal upset.
   * To prevent rheumatic fever or glomerulonephritis: unproven.
   * To avoid a follow-up consultation. Children receiving antibiotics for a sore throat are just as likely to reattend as those who do not. Antibiotics give an unrealistic expectation of cure. Review is often more appropriate than a prescription. The patient will return for a prescription every time his sore throat is as bad as the one you prescribed for.

- To reduce the duration of clinical symptoms. In 30% an antibiotic will reduce the duration of clinical symptoms by up to 48 hours.

2 . Tonsillectomy. Parents considering tonsillectomy and/or adenoidectomy should be informed of the normal size of tonsils in children and the expected frequency of respiratory infections as many have unrealistic expectations. Few are aware that there will be no reduction in the frequency of respiratory infections after surgery. Each year about 20 children die as a result of these operations.
Indications.
- Tuberculous cervical adenitis.
- Airways obstruction.
- Quinsy (not every case).
- Tonsillitis causing more than 3 weeks absence from school for 2 years. Check parents' reports against medical records and school health service records.
- Recurrent otitis media associated with tonsillitis.

3 . Adenoidectomy. See 'Ear, nose and throat'.

Diphtheria
Incidence. Rare in Britain.
Clinically. Corynebacterium diphtheria exotoxin causes local necrosis with an adherent pseudomembrane. The location of the pseudomembrane determines the clinical syndrome:
- Yellow membrane in nose. Coryza with serosanguineous discharge.
- Yellow membrane confined to tonsils. Mild sore throat, paralysed palate (nasal voice, dysphagia).
- Black membrane on tonsils and pharynx. 'Bullneck', low fever, systemic absorption of toxin causes hypotension, paralysis and myocarditis.
- Membrane on larynx. Stridor. Often need tracheostomy.
Management. If you suspect diphtheria give penicillin and antitoxin while waiting for the throat swab to be cultured.

Acute epiglottitis
Aetiology. Haemophilus influenzae infection causing massive swelling of the epiglottis.
Epidemiology. Age 2 to 6 years. Uncommon.

Clinically. Within a few hours of developing a sore throat and coryza the child is terrified, hot, toxic and drooling. He has inspiratory stridor, recession and holds his head in hyperextension to keep the airway clear. Cyanosis leads to respiratory arrest.

Management. Do not examine the throat as this may precipitate respiratory arrest. Accompany the child to hospital in case an emergency tracheostomy is necessary. Definitive treatment involves nasopharyngeal intubation and ampicillin or chloramphenicol. The illness lasts 7 days.

Differential diagnosis. See croup.

INFECTIONS OF THE LOWER RESPIRATORY TRACT

Laryngotracheitis (croup)

Aetiology. Inflammation of the larynx, trachea and bronchi caused by viruses (parainfluenza, RSV).

Epidemiology. Common from age 3 months to 3 years, commonest in the second year of life. Boys > girls.

Clinically. After a couple of days of coryza the child wakes at 2 am with a barking cough, a hoarse voice and a moderate fever. In mild cases there is mild intercostal recession, the respiratory rate is less than 40, and auscultation reveals a few scattered crackles and wheezes. In severe cases there is suprasternal retraction, stridor, tachypnoea >100 breaths per minute, tachycardia >150 beats per minute and the child is frightened and restless. Central cyanosis and exhaustion are signs of imminent respiratory arrest.

Management. Humidification in a cool room, minimal handling, drinks and paracetamol. Admit to hospital for humidified oxygen if the child does not settle within 1 hour, or if the parents are unable to cope, or if he is very breathless. Some need tracheostomy or ventilation. Of those admitted about 2% will die.

Complications. Viral bronchiolitis, secondary bacterial infection.

Differential diagnosis of stridor.

1. Croup.
2. Acute epiglottitis has a more rapid onset than croup, drooling is more marked and the cough is less prominent. Voice is not hoarse (vocal cords spared).
3. Foreign body in the larynx. Afebrile. Parents usually tell you the diagnosis.
4. Congenital idiopathic laryngeal stridor. 1 in 200 births. Intermittent mild stridor in a well baby. Spontaneous resolution.

5. Rarely: Allergic oedema; tracheomalacia; papilloma of the vocal cords; laryngospasm due to hypocalcaemia; tracheal compression from lymph nodes, goitre or abscess; diphtheria.

Bronchitis

Bronchitis and asthma are often indistinguishable in childhood. Classification based on the presence or absence of infection is meaningless since asthma is often precipitated by viral infections ('wheezy bronchitis'). Classification based on the reversibility of airways obstruction is confused by the reversible component of acute infections and the irreversible component of severe chronic asthma. A therapeutic trial of bronchodilators or steroids (covered by antibiotics) is a pragmatic solution. Passive or active inhalation of cigarette smoke can precipitate both conditions.

Bronchiolitis

Aetiology. Viral (RSV > parainfluenza). Bronchioles are blocked by submucosal oedema, mucus and sloughed epithelial cells.
Epidemiology. Affects 3% of infants. Males (3:2), winter epidemics.
Clinically. After a few days of coryza the child develops a fruity cough and wheeze. He drinks poorly. He will have a low fever, tachypnoea (50-100 breaths per minute), recession and hyperinflation. Auscultation reveals widespread fine crackles and expiratory wheeze. Heart failure is rare but is frequently suspected because the hyperinflated lungs push the liver down. Anoxia causes restlessness and sometimes cyanosis. Dehydration and exhaustion and cyanosis are signs of impending cardiorespiratory collapse. Apnoea can occur in younger infants. In uncomplicated cases the illness lasts about one week.
Management.
• Treat mild cases at home with humidification if the parents are confident and the CxR is normal.
• Give antibiotics if the fever rises suggesting bacterial superinfection.
• Many infants will need admission for humidified oxygen and i.v. fluids. 2% require ventilation.
• Drugs used for asthma do not help.
Prognosis. 1% die. Up to 50% have recurrent wheeze for years, and half of these have classical asthma.

Differential diagnosis of first episode of wheezing.
- Bronchiolitis.
- Asthma and bronchitis in infants are indistinguishable from bronchiolitis.
- Pneumonia causes more fever.
- Aspirated foreign body alters the CxR.
- Croup causes stridor and few chest signs.
- Whooping cough causes few chest signs and a marked lymphocytosis (WBC is normal in bronchiolitis).
- Congestive heart failure (Cardiomegaly on CxR).

Influenza

Virology. Orthomyxoviruses. Types A, B, C distinguished by the core S-antigen. Surface carries neuraminidase (N-antigen) and haemaglutinin (H-antigen). The N and H antigens undergo 'drift' and 'shift'. Immunity is strain specific.

Epidemiology. Transmitted by droplet. Type A causes epidemics and pandemics. Type B causes outbreaks in small communities. Type C occurs sporadically as a mild illness.

Clinically. 2-3 day incubation. Sudden malaise, headache, myalgia, fever, nausea, dry cough. Recover after 1 week. Complications: bacterial pneumonia (2%); otitis media (4%); rarely myocarditis, encephalomyelitis, influenza pneumonia, Reye's syndrome (with aspirin).

Treatment. Each autumn immunise vulnerable children with antigens of expected strain. Amantadine to contacts in closed communities.

Pneumonia

Aetiology.
- Neonatal pneumonias are usually bacterial: E.coli, S. pyogenes.
- After the neonatal period pneumonia is more commonly due to viruses (RSV, parainfluenza, influenza, adenovirus) than bacteria (Pneumococcus and Staphylococcus in pre-school children, Pneumococcus and Mycoplasma in school children).
- Adolescents, like adults, have more bacterial than viral pneumonias. Viral infections precede most bacterial pneumonias.

Epidemiology. 0.2% of children develop pneumonia each year. The incidence falls sharply with age. Predisposing factors: cystic fibrosis and impaired immunity.

Clinically.
- After a few days with a sore throat or runny nose the child develops a high fever and a worsening cough. Anorexia, vomiting, diarrhoea, headache and malaise are common. An older child may complain of pleuritic chest pain. Myalgia and arthralgia suggest mycoplasma.

- The child appears unwell with nasal flare, grunting respiration, tachypnoea and intercostal recession. Localising chest signs (dull percussion note, crackles and bronchial breathing) are often absent on first presentation.

Investigation. CxR and full blood count (FBC) for leucocytosis.

Management.
- Admit to hospital if the child is very unwell, or vomits medicines, or worsens on treatment or if fails to improve after 48 hours.
- Admit to hospital if the parents cannot cope
- Advise parents on fever control, warning signs (increasing tachypnoea, unable to drink) and expected course of the illness.
- Antibiotics should be prescribed. Expect recovery within one week of starting antibiotics. Repeat the CxR after recovery.

Complications.
- Death. Each year pneumonia kills 7 per 100,000 children and 80% of these are infants. All other respiratory infections together kill only half this number.
- Bronchiectasis.
- Lung abscess or empyema (S. aureus)
- Spread through the blood: meningitis (Haemophilus).

Whooping cough

Epidemiology. Every 2 to 3 years there is a summer epidemic of infections with Bordetella pertussis affecting 60,000 people and killing 10 to 15. There are 2,000 cases in non-epidemic years. Of those clinically affected 70% are under 6 years of age. Death is uncommon after infancy.

Clinically. After a 2 week incubation the child develops coryza, low fever and a dry cough. The cough starts to come in spasms terminated by a sharp gasp (the whoop) and a vomit. During severe bouts of coughing the child can suffer nosebleeds, subconjunctival haemorrhages, petechiae on the skin, hernias and a torn lingual frenulum. After a month the cough begins to settle. Auscultation reveals a few scattered coarse wheezes and crackles unless complications develop.

Complications. 1 in 5,000 die.
1. The infection damages ciliated respiratory epithelium and stimulates the production of sticky mucus. Mucus plugs and secondary infection commonly cause atelectasis, bronchitis and pneumonia. Bronchiectasis is rare because of antibiotic therapy.
2. Exhaustion, dehydration, alkalosis.
3. Apnoea in infants.
4. Pneumothorax, pneumomediastinum and subcutaneous emphysema (rare).
5. Cerebro-vascular accidents, encephalitis and convulsions (1 in 100,000).
Investigation. Lymphocytosis ≥ 15,000, with a relative neutropenia. Normal CxR before complications develop. Culture Bordetella from pernasal swab or cough plate, or demonstrate a rising titre of antibodies.
Differential diagnosis. See 'asthma'.
Treatment. Isolate at home while infectious (from 7 days after exposure until three weeks after the cough becomes paroxysmal). Parents should take it in turns to sleep near the child. Encourage fluids and avoid dry food that might cause coughing. Sleep face down to allow secretions to drain. Erythromycin kills the organism in the first week of infection but does not affect the illness. Admit if complications develop or to give the parents a rest.
Prevention. Immunise. Erythromycin to unimmunised contacts.

Bronchiectasis
Aetiology.
Inherited
• Cystic fibrosis. Autosomal recessive. 1/2,000 live births are homozygotes. See 'Gastrointestinal tract'.
• Kartagener's syndrome. Probably autosomal recessive. Abnormal cilial function. Affects 1/40,000. Bronchiectasis, sinusitis, situs inversus.
• Hypogammaglobulinaemia. Very rare.
Acquired (usually before school age). Rare.
• Pneumonia especially following pertussis or measles.
• Inhaled foreign body.
• Tuberculosis.
Pathology. Obstruction of bronchi with distal collapse and infection. Heals with dilated bronchi and cystic spaces.
Clinically. Chronic or recurrent productive cough. Haemoptysis (50%). Pigeon or barrel chest. Harrison's sulcus. Auscultation reveals coarse crackles and occasional coarse wheeze. Cyanosis, clubbing, and oedema in advanced disease.

Complications.

Common:

- atelectasis, pneumonia, reversible obstructive airways disease (asthma).
- sinusitis.
- short stature.
- anaemia,

Terminal:

- cor pulmonale.

Uncommon:

- pneumothorax, empyema, bronchopleural fistula, massive haemoptysis.
- amyloidosis.
- brain abscess.

Investigations.

- CxR initially normal but cysts and areas of collapse and fibrosis. eventually develop.
- Sputum culture. Initially pneumococcus and H. influenzae. Later S. aureus, Klebsiella, Pseudomonas, Aspergillus fumigatus.
- Sweat test to confirm cystic fibrosis.
- FBC and immunoglobulin levels to screen for immune deficiency.
- Bronchogram if localised, resectable, disease is suspected.

Treatment. Bronchiectasis is best managed in specialist centres. GPs should support the family and manage milder chest infections.

1. Immunise against pertussis, measles, tuberculosis and influenza.
2. Encourage regular physiotherapy by the parents or self physiotherapy by older children. Percussion, postural drainage, forced expiration ('huffing').
3. Antibiotics for chest infections. Ampicillin is first choice.
4. Treat coexisting asthma.

Prognosis. Inherited bronchiectasis has a worse prognosis than acquired disease. 50% of patients with cystic fibrosis reach age 20.

Lung abscess

Aetiology.

1. Pneumonia (especially Klebsiella and S. aureus).
2. Aspiration of a foreign body.
3. Bronchiectasis.
4. Tuberculosis.
5. Very rarely: septicaemia, cavitating neoplasm, trauma, sequestered lobe.

Clinically. Malaise, fever, weight loss, cough, haemoptysis, clubbing. Chest clear on auscultation. See bronchiectasis for complications.

Management.
- CxR.
- Refer for further investigation (bronchoscopy, bronchogram) and treatment (antibiotics, surgery).
- Usually resolve completely with antibiotics.

ASTHMA

Aetiology. A condition characterized by reversible airway obstruction. The basic defect is hyper-reactivity of the bronchi to specific allergens (IgE mediated) and non-specific stimuli. The reaction tends to occlude the lumen of the bronchi by contraction of the encircling smooth muscle, mucosal oedema and the production of excessive amounts of sticky mucus. Allergens may be inhaled (house dust mite proteins) or ingested (tartrazine). Non-specific stimuli include viral respiratory tract infections, cold air, smoke, exertion, hyperventilation and emotion.

Epidemiology. 10% of children and 1% of adults are affected. Familial and associated with eczema, allergic rhinitis, urticaria and dermographism. Increasingly common among urban dwellers in developed nations.

Clinically. Tight feeling in the chest and exhaling. Productive cough and wheeze. Worse at night and in the early morning ('morning dip').
- The most mildly affected develop a persistent cough after viral respiratory infections (wheezy bronchitis).
- Moderately severe asthma causes episodic symptoms. During an attack the child has difficulty talking. His chest is hyperinflated with intercostal recession and tachypnoea. Wheezes and crackles on auscultation. Tachycardia and paradoxical hypotension on inspiration. Hypoxic restlessness, cyanosis or exhaustion are warnings of impending cardio-respiratory collapse.
- Severe asthma with almost continual symptoms is uncommon in childhood.

Investigation.
- Peak expiratory flow rate (PEFR) is essential for diagnosis and monitoring. A 20% change in PEF during a 24 hour period or after exercise or after bronchodilator is diagnostic of asthma. In some cases reversibility can only be demonstrated after a steroid trial.
- Spirometry confirms airways obstruction if the ratio of Forced Expiratory Volume in 1 second (FEV_1) to Vital Capacity (VC) is less than 75%.
- CxR is useful to exclude other diagnoses and check for complications.

- Eosinophilia, high levels of IgE precipitins and skin sensitivity tests may support a diagnosis of asthma but seldom affect management. Skin sensitivity to an allergen does not prove bronchial sensitivity, only a trial of exclusion and rechallenge can verify this. Challenge with inhaled allergen is a specific research tool (can cause respiratory arrest).

Management. Response to therapy improves after infancy. By the age of 2 years asthma can be controlled with currently available therapy if it is used correctly. Good inhaler technique and, in persistent asthma, regular usage of inhaled anti-inflammatory therapy are fundamental to good asthma control and require regular and repeated assessment. Cigarette smoking (active or passive), poor compliance and inefficient use of inhalers are the commonest causes of treatment failure.

Prescribing.

- Bronchodilators can be used alone for intermittent mild attacks: beta-adrenergic agonists such as salbutamol. anti-cholinergic ipratropium bromide. Syrups (for toddlers), pressurized aerosols with spacer devices (age 4), dry powder devices (age 6). Nebulised bronchodilators are best used under close medical supervision during severe attacks. Overdependence on nebulisers by parents who do not fully understand the indications for steroid therapy is thought to contribute to the increasing incidence of asthma-related deaths in children.
- Controlled-release oral theophyllines may be useful in the treatment of nocturnal asthma but theraputic levels may cause unacceptable side effects including nausea and hyperactivity. Intravenous theophyllines may be useful in severe attacks.
- Anti-inflammatory agents. Inhaled sodium cromoglycate or steroid should be used regularly if bronchodilators are needed more than a few times each week. Nebuliser delivery of inhaled steroid is often ineffective.
- Oral corticosteroid. Prednisolone should be given at the onset of any severe attack (2 mg/kg up to 40 mg daily). Chronic severe asthma sometimes responds only to continuous oral steroid.

Other therapy.

- Physiotherapy by the parents of toddlers helps clear mucus.
- Obsessive cleaning of the child's room and foam pillows are scarcely better than 'normal middle class' ideals of cleanliness and furnishing.
- Be sure that the child is allergic to its pet (exclusion for months then rechallenge) before you order its slaughter.
- Avoid passive or active smoking.
- Activities, including sports, as tolerated.
- Career choice should avoid recognised allergens.

Differential diagnosis of recurrent or persistent cough and wheeze.
1. Normal response to successive upper respiratory infections.
2. Asthma, bronchitis, recurrent bronchiolitis are virtually indistinguishable. Try a therapeutic trial of bronchodilator or oral prednisolone.
3. Whooping cough.
4. Bronchiectasis (Sweat test).
5. Inhaled foreign body (abnormal CxR).
6. Cardiac failure. Cardiomegaly on CxR.
7. Tuberculosis.
8. Nervous 'tic'.
9. Other causes are worthy of case reports, e.g. immune deficiency.

ASPIRATION
1. **Gastric contents** may be aspirated by infants requiring intensive care especially if they have a tracheo-oesophageal fistula. Children with dysphagia, coma, oesophageal reflux or vomiting (especially with the whoop of pertussis) can aspirate. The acidic fluid causes haemorrhagic necrosis, bronchospasm and acidosis. The child is cyanosed and may stop breathing. Cough and wheeze. Crackles over affected lobe (usually right lower lobe is worst affected). Admit for bronchial lavage, antibiotics and ventilation. In the ambulance suck out the back of the throat, give oxygen and intravenous saline, lie in the best position to drain the affected lobe. High mortality.
2. **Discrete foreign bodies** (peanuts or toys) are inhaled by older infants and toddlers. Parents often know what has happened. A foreign body (FB) in the larynx causes tachypnoea, cough and stridor. An FB in a bronchus causes tachypnoea, cough, localised wheeze and crackles. The CxR shows obstructive emphysema or collapse distal to a bronchial FB. Needs bronchoscopic removal.
3. **Household cleaners and solvents.**

NEOPLASIA
Benign (very rare): pulmonary hamartoma, bronchial adenoma, tracheobronchial papilloma.
Malignant primary (very rare): bronchogenic carcinoma. Sarcoma.
Malignant secondary (uncommon): leukaemia, sarcomata (Wilm's, neuroblastoma, osteosarcoma, Ewing's).

11. EAR NOSE AND THROAT

EARACHE

Outer ear. Pain worse on moving the pinna. Otitis externa, a boil in the ear canal, trauma, impacted wax, foreign bodies.

Middle ear. Acute otitis media. Glue ear. Chronic suppurative otitis media (rare in children).

Tympanic membrane.

* Myringitis bullosa. Painful vesicles on the tympanic membrane (TM) associated with mycoplasma or viral respiratory infections.
* Traumatic perforation.

Referred pain. Pharynx, teeth, cervical adenopathy.

Otitis externa

Incidence. A GP sees 15 affected children each year.

Aetiology.

* Skin disease: eczema, seborrhoeic dermatitis.
* Damp: swimming, ear syringing, ear drops, middle ear discharge.
* Trauma caused by finger nail, cotton bud, or foreign body.
* Infections: boil, cellulitis, candida. Secondary infection often follows one of the other causes of otitis externa.

Clinically. Earache worse on moving the pinna. Discharge.

Treatment. Dry mopping. Topical antibiotics, antifungals, or steroids. Paracetamol. Careful drying after swimming.

Foreign bodies

Common. Unless an object can be removed first time - leave it to an ENT surgeon.

Acute suppurative otitis media

Incidence. Affects 20% of pre-school children each year. 50% of all children have been affected by age 10. Peak incidence age 4 to 8, unusual after age 10. The average GP will see 75 cases each year.

Risk factors: atopy, smoking household, social classes 4 and 5. Chronic infection of adenoids or tonsils or sinuses. Cleft palate.

Aetiology. Infection of the middle ear mucosa. Usually viral. 90% of severe cases and 10% of mild cases are bacterial (Pneumococcus, Haemophilus influenzae, Strep. pyogenes, B. catarrhalis).

Clinically. During an episode of coryza or pharyngitis the child develops earache, deafness, tinnitus and fever. If the TM perforates, pus discharges and the pain subsides. In mild cases the TM is injected or dull red, in severe cases the TM is red and bulging. Air insufflation shows reduced TM mobility.

Investigations. Tympanocentesis is seldom necessary. Cultures of swabs of the throat or aural discharge are seldom helpful.

Treatment.
- Paracetamol for fever and pain.
- Dry mopping any discharge helps prevent otitis externa. No swimming until the perforation has healed.
- Antibiotics are indicated if the earache is severe, or the child is unwell, or the drum is discharging, or within 3 months of otitis media. Amoxycillin (under age 5) or penicillin (after age 5).
- Topical or oral decongestants or antihistamines do not help.
- Myringotomy relieves pain but is rarely necessary.

Complications. 10% develop glue ear, 1% develop chronic suppurative otitis media. Rarely mastoiditis, meningitis, cerebral abscess.

Secretory otitis media (glue ear)

Incidence. At least 5% of children have glue ear at any one time.

At risk. Age 2 – 8, allergic rhinitis, sinusitis, adenoid hypertrophy. Down's Syndrome (70%), cleft palate (100%).

Aetiology. Eustacian insufficiency results in resorption of air in middle ear and a sticky exudate. Often preceded by acute otitis media.

Clinically. Mild earache, well, afebrile. Parents may notice deafness or deteriorating speech. Older children may have learning difficulties or behaviour problems. TM dull yellow and immobile on air insufflation.

Investigation. Pure tone audiograms show impaired hearing, especially of low frquencies. Tympanometry is diagnostic.

Management. Tell the parents the expected course of the condition.
- Suggest that the child watches the lips of anyone speaking to him and sits at the front of the class.
- Review monthly with pure tone audiometry.
- Refer to ENT surgeon if the child has learning difficulties or if the condition lasts more than 3 months. Myringotomy and grommets restore hearing sufficiently to permit learning. Adenoidectomy may be performed at the same time. Ear plugs when swimming. Grommets last 3-12 months, and are not replaced if hearing remains adequate.

Prognosis. Uncommon after puberty. Seldom causes permanent hearing damage.

FACIAL PAIN
- Dental pain.
- Otitis media.
- Cellulitis.
- Sinusitis.
- Migraine and trigeminal neuralgia.
- Mumps parotitis.

Sinusitis
Incidence. Classical sinusitis is uncommon before adolescence, but inflammation of the mucosa lining the paranasal sinuses with blockage of the ostia and accumulation of fluid is common.

Risk factors. Allergic or vasomotor rhinitis, fractured nose, dental abscess, deviated nasal septum, chronic tonsilitis or adcnoiditis.

Clinically. During a coryzal illness the child develops facial pain and a purulent, bloodstained nasal discharge. Fever, toxaemia and facial swelling are uncommon and suggest a dental abscess or cellulitis. Some children notice a post-nasal drip and loss of the senses of smell and taste.

Investigations.
- Culture of nasal discharge is often sterile. Sometimes: H. influenzae, Pneumococcus, S. aureus, B. catarrhalis, anaerobes.
- Sinus X-ray may reveal mucosal swelling, polyps and a fluid level.
- X-ray of facial bones and teeth in atypical cases.

Treatment. Avoid swimming and flying.
  - Paracetamol and steam inhalation.
  - Ephedrine nose drops for up to 5 days (oral decongestants do not help).
  - Antibiotics.
  - Refer children with atypical cases or after treatment has failed. Antral lavage is rarely needed and antrostomy is to be avoided in growing bones.

DEAFNESS
Speech uses the frequencies 400 to 4,000 Hz.

Hearing threshold > 90 decibels (dB) = total deafness.

> 60 dB	= cannot hear normal speech.
> 30 dB	= difficulty with group conversations.
> 20 dB	= retarded language development.
≤ 20 dB	= normal hearing.

Incidence. 1/1,000 live births are very deaf (mostly sensorineural deafness of which 50% is inherited). 5% of 7 year olds and 1% of 10 year olds have significant deafness (mostly due to glue ear).

Aetiology.
1. Genetic (sensorineural):
   - Isolated defect.
   - Part of a syndrome.
2. Non-genetic (sensorineural):
   - Congenital rubella or cytomegalovirus infection.
   - Neonatal jaundice, anoxia, or trauma.
   - Mumps or measles.
   - Meningitis or encephalitis.
   - Gentamycin overdose.
   - Head injury.
   - Noise (disco music).
3. Non-genetic (conductive):
   - Otitis media and glue ear.
   - Middle ear or external ear malformation.
   - Middle ear damage including perforation of the TM.
   - Obstruction of the external ear: wax, foreign body, meatal stenosis.
   - Otosclerosis.
4. Cortical deafness.
5. Hysteria.

Screening.
- Neonate: turns towards a voice; auditory response cradle.
- Infant up to 8 months old: distraction testing (turns to sound); questionnaire for parents.
- After age 2: In word-object tests the observer whispers the name of a test object and the child points to it (McCormack). In a conditioning test the child is asked to perform a simple task on hearing a sound. Simple equipment is available to produce standardized sounds or measure the intensity of a tester's whispers.

Assessment.
- Otoscopic examination.
- The Rinné test uses a tuning fork (512 Hz) to determine whether air conduction is better than bone. Difficult to apply in childhood.
- Audiometry: speech (before age 5) or pure tone audiograms (after by age 5).
- Tympanometry. An earpiece bounces sound off the TM. The compliance of the TM at different pressures can distinguish between a blocked Eustacian tube, fluid in the middle ear, a perforated TM, and a scarred TM or ossicular dislocation.
- Occasional children will need auditory evoked potentials, skull X-rays and computerized tomography (CAT) scans.

Treatment.
- Advise family and teachers to speak clearly when facing the child.
- Support groups.
- Special educational provision including speech therapy, and training in sign language and lip reading.
- Hearing aids.
- Special aids such as radio transmitters for teachers in schools for the deaf.
- Surgery. Glue ear may require myringotomy, grommets and adenoidectomy. Reconstructive surgery may help some conditions.
- Employment advice and training.
- Genetic counselling.

Prognosis. Glue ear usually resolves in adolescence. Sensorineural deafness is almost always permanent and may deteriorate. Severe deafness can isolate a child especially if there are additional handicaps.

Chronic adenoid hypertrophy

Incidence. Common, especially from age 2 to 8 years.
Clinically.
- Persistent purulent nasal discharge and nasal obstruction sufficient to disturb sleep and make eating difficult. Nocturnal hypoxaemia or sleep apnoea can cause daytime drowsiness. Snoring that wakes the parents but leaves an alert child the next day is their problem not his.
- Recurrent or persistent glue ear.

Investigation. Demonstrate by lateral X-ray of the neck. If a prolonged course of antibiotics fails, try cromoglycate or beclomethasone nose drops before referral for a surgical opinion.

Indications for adenoidectomy.
1. Chronic severe nasal obstruction unresponsive to medical treatment, especially if causing sleep apnoea.
2. Otitis media causing school absence more than 3 times each year for more than 2 years.
3. Speech delay associated with hearing loss due to glue ear and chronic adenoid hypertrophy.
4. Tuberculous cervical adenitis.

Contraindications. Serious nasal escape may develop after adenoidectomy in children with short or cleft palates or bifid uvula.

STRIDOR
See 'Respiratory disease'.

NASAL DISCHARGE
- Coryza.
- Rhinitis.
- Foreign body in the nose.
- Rare causes: CSF leak.

Rhinitis
Incidence. 20% of children have non-viral rhinitis. Atopic children and families.
Aetiology.
- Usually allergic: seasonal (hayfever), perennial.
- Sometimes vasomotor rhinitis.
Clinically. Sneezing and itching. Clear or purulent nasal discharge. Swelling of nasal mucosa. Conjunctivitis.
Investigation.
- Specific sensitivity on inhalation challenge is a research procedure.
- Atopy is suggested by eosinophilia, high IgE.
Treatment.
- Avoid allergen. Desensitizing injections help those with a single seasonal allergen.
- Antihistamines. Cromoglycate nose drops or steroid nose drops. Oral or intramuscular steroid in severe cases.
- Excision of chronic nasal polyps or cautery of mucosa.

NOSEBLEEDS
Aetiology.
- Commonly due to nose picking or coryza.
- Occasionally due to trauma, telangiectasia, bleeding tendency.
- Rarely due to neoplasm or hypertension.
Clinically. Usually bleeding from Little's area on the anterior part of the nasal septum.
Treatment.
- Bleeding from Littles's area: pinch the end of the nose, silver nitrate cautery for recurrent bleeding.
- Bleeding from the back of the nose: nasal pack or Brighton balloon. Refer if this fails.

12. TEETH MOUTH AND JAWS

SORE MOUTH

Baby and young child
- Teething may cause discomfort but nothing else.
- Dental caries
- Infection: tonsillitis, mouth ulcers (herpes gingivostomatitis, hand foot and mouth syndrome, Candidosis).
- Eruption cysts. see 'Disorders of eruption'
- Trauma

Teenager
- Dental caries and gingivitis
- Apthous ulcers
- Impacted wisdom teeth. See 'Disorders of eruption'.
- Angioneurotic oedema
- Cold sores
- Sinusitis
- Trauma

Dental caries and gingivitis
Aetiology. Dietary polysaccharides stick to teeth (plaque) and bacteria convert them to acid which decalcifies the enamel and destroys the organic matrix.

Incidence. 50% of children have dental caries by age 5, and the average 12 year old has 3 decayed/missing/filled teeth.

Prevention.
- Fluoridation of drinking water (1 part per million) halves the incidence of dental caries. A daily fluoride tablet can be as effective as water fluoridation, but compliance is seldom perfect. Fluoride toothpaste is less effective.
- Reducing the frequency of eating refined carbohydrate that feeds the bacteria causing caries.
- Regular dental checks. Reducing the destruction of sound tooth to a minimum when drilling to insert fillings.
- Careful brushing of teeth and gums.

Oral trauma
Apply pressure to stop haemorrhage. Look for jaw fracture and loose or cracked teeth. If teeth are missing consider whether they could have been inhaled. Dislodged teeth can be kept clean and warm in the mouth of an older child (or milk) and reimplanted by a dentist.

MOUTH ULCERS
- **Viral infections**: herpetic gingivostomatitis, hand foot and mouth disease (coxsackie virus), and AIDS.
- **Candidosis**.
- **Apthous ulcers**
  10% of teenagers suffer from recurrent oral ulcers, but the frequency declines with age. The aetiology is unknown. These ulcers are painful, frequently get infected and last about two weeks. Each ulcer is round and sharply defined with a collar of erythema. Adcortyl in orabase relieves pain.
- **Traumatic**.
- **Allergy and drug toxicity**.
- Rare causes: anaemia, agranulocytosis, Stevens-Johnson syndrome, Vincent's infection, AIDS, Kawasaki syndrome, B_{12} and folate deficiency.

MALFORMATION

Cleft lip and palate
Incidence. 1:300 births. 1:10 have another malformation.
Aetiology. Usually idiopathic. Sometimes familial or associated with intrauterine exposure to drugs.
Pathology. The upper lip and palate are formed by fusion of a midline fronto-nasal process growing down to fuse with a maxillary process on either side. Failure of this process can result in a unilateral cleft lip (20%), bilateral cleft lip (4%), cleft upper lip and palate (50%), and cleft palate (25%).
Clinically. A cleft lip causes little functional problem but causes severe parental distress and can lead to rejection of the child. A cleft palate interferes with sucking, and is associated with otitis media, speech impairment and malocclusion.
Management. A baby with a cleft palate needs to be fed with a dropper or spoon until a prosthetic plate can be fitted to separate the mouth from the nose. Repair a cleft lip at 2-6 months and a cleft palate at 1 year. Even after a definitive repair the child may need speech therapy.

Malocclusion
The anterior lower teeth normally lie touching and slightly posterior to the upper teeth when the jaw is closed. The posterior upper teeth normally close on to the lower teeth. In malocclusion this pattern is lost for some or all of the teeth. An 'open bite' interferes with chewing and may lead to temporomandibular joint arthritis in adult life. Mild malocclusions are very common.

Aetiology.
1. Finger- or dummy-sucking displaces the upper anterior teeth forward. Usually resolves in later childhood when the habit stops.
2. Premature extraction of carious primary teeth allows adjacent teeth to drift.
3. A small jaw leads to dental crowding. In extreme cases, such as Pierre-Robin syndrome, micrognathia may cause sleep apnoea (tongue obstructs airway) and feeding difficulties.
4. The upper and lower dental arches, or the maxilla and mandible themselves, may be misaligned. This is often familial.

Management. Mild malocclusions do not require treatment. Moderate malocclusions may require orthodontic treatment or dental extractions. Severe malocclusions may require maxillofacial surgery.

Defective teeth
1. **Missing teeth.** 25% of caucasians do not have third molars. If a lot of teeth are missing consider ectodermal dysplasia and related syndromes.
2. **Small teeth.**
3. **Malformed teeth.** Enamel defects occur in 1/2,000 children. Some syndromes include dental defects (osteogenesis imperfecta).
4. **Discoloured teeth.** Tetracyclines.

Disorders of eruption
The first tooth usually erupts at 6 months. All 20 deciduous teeth are present by age 5 when the first permanent tooth erupts. By age 15 there are 28 permanent teeth, but the 4 wisdom teeth may need another 10 years to come through.
1. **Natal teeth** present at birth should be removed if loose.
2. **Delayed eruption of all the teeth** may be idiopathic or associated with hypothyroidism, Down's syndrome, rickets, congenital syphilis or cleidocranial dysostosis.
3. **Isolated delayed eruption** may be due to trauma to a growing tooth, crowding or local infection.
5. **Extra teeth** are common.
6. **Eruption cysts.** Incidence declines with age. A painful bluish swelling over an erupting tooth. Incise after applying local anaesthetic gel.
7. **Wisdom teeth.** Impacted wisdom teeth may cause pain. Once the tooth erupts the gum flap is prone to infection resulting in a painful cellulitis. Saline mouth washes to remove debris. Antibiotics for the cellulitis.

13. CARDIOVASCULAR SYSTEM

THE INNOCENT CARDIAC MURMUR
- Symptomless.
- Systolic.
- Short.
- Soft (no thrill).
- Small area.
- Sitting or deep inspiration makes the murmur quieter.
- Second sound splits normally in the pulmonary area into the sound of aortic valve closure followed by the sound of pulmonic valve closure. First sound is single because the mitral and tricuspid valves close together. No ejection clicks.
- The character and rhythm of the carotid pulse is normal and all peripheral pulses are normal.
- The precordial impulse is normal.
- The ECG, CxR and echocardiogram are normal.

There are two common types of benign murmur:
- **Flow murmur**. Soft, low pitched, systolic murmur at the lower left sternal border. Intensity varies with posture. May be quite loud when the cardiac output is increased such as during a febrile illness.
- **Venous hum**. Continuous murmur at the right upper sternal border or neck. Disappears when the child is supine.

HYPERTENSION
The mean blood pressure (bp) increases from 95/55 in infancy to 115/70 in adolescence. The corresponding 95th percentiles are 115/80 in infancy and 140/90 in adolescence. The level of hypertension that requires treatment in childhood is unknown. Most paediatricians would treat a diastolic >90 before age 13, and a diastolic >100 after age 13.

Aetiology. Secondary hypertension becomes commoner the younger the child and the higher the bp. 50% of cases after age 13 are idiopathic, of the remainder:
- **80% Renal parenchymal**: Chronic pyelonephritis, hydronephrosis, tumours, chronic glomerulonephritis.
- **10% Renovascular** (renal artery stenosis).
- **10% Others**: coarctation of the aorta, excess corticosteroids (C.A.H., Cushings, therapeutic), primary hyperaldosteronism, phaeochromocytoma, neuroblastoma, thyrotoxicosis, hyper-calcaemia, raised intracranial pressure.

Symptoms.
- Of renal causes (haematuria, dysuria, polyuria). Of endocrine causes (heat intolerance, flushing, diarrhoea).
- Of malignant hypertension (headache, chest pain, fits, drowsiness).

Signs.
- Signs of malignant hypertension (retinal haemorrhages, papilloedema, heart failure, encephalopathy).
- Signs of aetiology (renal or adrenal masses, renal artery bruit, enlarged bladder, goitre, radio-femoral delay, neurofibromatosis).

Investigation.
- Renal causes. Urine for blood, protein, microscopy, culture. Ultrasound kidneys, IVP. Blood for creatinine. Renal angiogram.
- Endocrine causes. Serum thyroxine, Ca^{2+}, Na^+, K^+, Cl^-, HCO_3^-. 24 hour urine for cortisol/VMA. Renal vein renin, aldosterone, noradrenaline.
- Hypertensive damage. CxR.

Treatment. Antihypertensive drugs. Surgery if indicated.

Prognosis. 30% become normotensive without therapy.

CHEST PAIN IN CHILDHOOD

- Pleurisy (pneumonia, Bornholm disease, pneumothorax).
- Chest wall problem: fractured rib, myalgia, muscle strain, osteochondritis.
- Oesophagitis.
- Psychological (hyperventilation).
- Pericarditis.
- Heart muscle disease: myocarditis, HOCM.
- Congenital heart disease: tetralogy of Fallot.
- Coronary artery disease (see heart failure).

ACUTE MYOCARDITIS

- Viral infection (Coxsackie B) is the commonest cause in the UK.
- Other: bacteraemia (legionella), toxic (cytotoxic drugs, diphtheria), immune (rheumatic fever, SLE).

Epidemiology. Uncommon. Epidemics of Coxsackie B infection in hospital nurseries, otherwise sporadic.

Clinically.
- Infant suddenly becomes anorexic, lethargic, hot, tachypnoeic, cyanosed and shocked. Cardiomegaly and hepatomegaly develop quickly. 75% die with heart block, arrhythmias or heart failure.
- Older children are less affected, and 90% recover rapidly and completely.

Investigation. Blood culture, viral titres, ASOT, throat swab (diphtheria), cardiac enzymes (elevated), ECG, CxR (often normal), Echocardiogram. Endomyocardial biopsy.

Treatment. Bed rest, oxygen, digoxin/diuretics/vasodilators, prednisolone and azathioprine. Avoid exertion until ECG normal.

CHRONIC MYOCARDITIS
Rare. Affects 10% of children with acute myocarditis. Presents as dilated cardiomyopathy.

PERICARDITIS
Incidence. Uncommon.
Aetiology.
- **Usually:** Cryptogenic, post viral (Coxsackie B) or post cardiac surgery (after 25% of operations).
- **Occasionally.** Purulent (S. aureus, H. influenzae, meningo-coccus). Tuberculous. Rheumatic fever. Collagen diseases. Leukaemic infiltration. Radiation. Cytotoxic drugs. Uraemia.

Clinically. Pain in the left chest, relieved on sitting forwards. High fever suggests purulent pericarditis. Breathlessness and dry cough as pericardial effusion collects. Pericardial rub. Cardiac tamponade when the effusion is tense (raised JVP, hepatomegaly, crackles in the lungs, reduced blood pressure with pulsus paradoxus).

Investigation. Echocardiogram shows effusions. CxR is normal until a massive effusion shows as a globular heart. Pericardiocentesis to exclude haemopericardium or septic pericarditis. Cardiac enzymes normal.

Treatment. Bed rest. Aspirin. Prednisolone for resistant cases. Purulent pericarditis needs antibiotics and surgical drainage. Pericardiocentesis for cardiac tamponade.

Prognosis. Usually recover completely. Rarely develop constrictive pericarditis with marked right heart failure and need pericardectomy .

HEART FAILURE IN INFANCY

In the UK heart failure in children usually occurs in the first 6 months of life as a consequence of congenital heart disease.
Aetiology listed by age of onset:
Week 1: hypoplasia of the left heart, transposition of the great arteries > birth asphyxia, hypocalcaemia, hypoglycaemia. Patent ductus arteriosus (PDA) is a common cause in premature babies.

- Week 2-4: coarctation of the aorta > myocarditis.
- Month 2-3: VSD, PDA.
- Month 3+: Coarctation of the aorta, tetralogy of Fallot.

Clinically. Infants present with tachycardia (>160), tachypnoea (>60) and cough. Later hepatomegaly (>2 cm below the costal margin) and excessive weight gain despite feeding poorly (>28 g or 1 oz per day). Very late signs are failure to thrive, pretibial oedema, wheezes and crackles heard in the lungs, cyanosis.

HEART FAILURE AFTER INFANCY

Aetiology.
Usually:
- Cryptogenic dilated cardiomyopathy.
- HOCM.

Sometimes:
- Congenital heart disease (only 10% of cases start after infancy).
- Valvular heart disease: congenital > SBE > rheumatic.
- Specific heart muscle disease. Myocarditis, storage diseases, muscular dystrophy, Freidrich's ataxia.

Occasionally:
- Coronary artery disease: accelerated atherosclerosis in familial hypercholesterolaemia, vasculitis (Kawasaki disease).
- Arrhythmias and heart block.
- High output failure due to arteriovenous malformations.
- Hypertension.

Clinically. Present with breathlessness on exertion. Cyanosis, finger clubbing, and growth retardation are late signs.

Treatment. Diuretics, digoxin, vasodilators, adrenergic inotropes. Corrective surgery is seldom indicated after infancy. Cardiac transplantation.

DILATED CARDIOMYOPATHY
Usually cryptogenic, sometimes follows myocarditis. Dilated left ventricle on echocardiogram. Virtually 100% mortality 5 years after diagnosis.

HYPERTROPHIC OBSTRUCTIVE CARDIOMYOPATHY
Incidence. Uncommon. Age 10-20. Usually familial (autosomal dominant with incomplete penetrance). Sometimes sporadic. Occasionally part of a syndrome (Friedreich's ataxia). Girls = boys.

Pathology. The myocardium is thickened. This reduces and narrows the outflow tract. On exertion the stiff ventricle fills incompletely during diastole (reduced cardiac output), coronary perfusion during diastole is impaired by the high end diastolic pressure (angina), and ventricular arrhythmias are common (syncope, sudden death).

Clinically. Breathless on exertion > angina > syncope. Jerky pulse, prominent apex beat with triple impulse. S4 (extra sound before S1). Ejection systolic murmur best heard medial to the apex beat, reduced by squatting and increased by valsalva.

Investigations. CxR is normal. ECG: left ventricle hypertrophy. Echocardiogram shows a hypertrophied interventricular septum. Cardiac catheter demonstrates the degree of outflow tract obstruction.

Treatment.
- Avoid competitive sport.
- ß-blockers or verapamil reduce exercise-related tachycardia and improve ventricular filling during diastole and coronary blood flow.
- Amiodarone for atrial fibrillation. Digoxin is contraindicated.
- Warfarin once paroxsymal atrial tachycardias develop (to prevent systemic emboli).
- Septal resection if medical treatment fails (10% operative mortality).

Prognosis. Infants with HOCM often die with heart failure except for the infants of diabetic mothers of whom 10% have HOCM that resolves in infancy. Children with HOCM have a 30% 10-year survival.

RHEUMATIC FEVER

Incidence. 3/100,000 children in UK. 1000/100,000 children in Northern India. Age 4-14 years. Girls = boys, but girls develop more valvular disease.

Pathology. Cross sensitivity between Group A streptococci and connective tissue results in diffuse and focal inflammation. Carditis (60%), pleurisy (10%), peritonitis (10%). Endocarditis causes valve stenosis or incompetence.

Diagnosis. Evidence of previous streptococcal infection (ASOT, throat swab, scarlatina) with 2 major criteria, or 1 major with 2 minor criteria.

Major criteria:
- Significant heart murmur (mitral or aortic regurgitation, mitral stenosis).
- Carditis: cardiomegaly (heart failure or pericardial effusion), cardiac failure or pericarditis (10%).
- Major arthritis (50%).
- Chorea (5%).
- Erythema marginatum (5%).
- Rheumatic nodules (5%).

Minor criteria: Fever (90%), ESR >20 (95%), prolonged PR interval (85%), arthralgia (90%).

Investigations. Anaemia and leucocytosis. Echocardiography to assess cardiomegaly (heart failure has a poor prognosis but pericardial effusions usually resolve).

Treatment.

- Primary prevention. Penicillin does not reduce the incidence of rheumatic fever after sore throats.
- Secondary prevention. Prophylactic Penicillin V until age 20 (or 40 if valves affected) reduces the incidence of recurrent attacks of rheumatic fever from 70% to 5%, and prevents further valve damage.
- Treatment of acute episode. Bed rest and aspirin for carditis or arthritis. Penicillin. Digoxin and diuretics for heart failure. Prednisolone may improve survival in acute attacks.
- Treatment of chronic valve disease. Cover surgery or dental care with a non-penicillin antibiotic. Warfarin if atrial arrhythmias develop. Mitral valvotomy for severe stenosis in childhood. Valve replacement in symptomatic adults.

Prognosis. Acute attacks have a 2% mortality from carditis. 30% develop valve disease (isolated mitral stenosis > mitral stenosis and incompetence > aortic regurgitation).

PULMONARY HYPERTENSION
- **Congenital heart disease** with a shunt allowing increased pulmonary arterial blood flow (VSD, ASD, TGV)
- **Hypoxia** (altitude, chronic upper airway obstruction, chronic obstructive lung disease)
- **Obstructive lesions of the left heart** causing pulmonary venous hypertension with subsequent arterial hypertension (mitral stenosis).
- **Pulmonary thromboembolism** by multiple small emboli (ventriculovenous drains for hydrocephalus).
- **Idiopathic** (may be familial)

Pathology. Chronic pulmonary hypertension causes intimal and medial hypertrophy of pulmonary arterioles. This increases pulmonary vascular resistance and increases the hypertension. Moderate arteriolar changes are reversed by removing the cause of the hypertension.

Signs. Left parasternal heave. Loud pulmonary component and reduced splitting of the second heart sound as the valve is slammed shut by the high arterial pressure. Early systolic click at the left sternal edge as the pulmonic valve opens.

Investigations. ECG, CxR and echocardiogram may suggest right ventricular hypertrophy.

CONGENITAL HEART DISEASE

Incidence. Congenital heart disease occurs in 1% of live births. Bicuspid aortic valve occurs in another 1% and may cause problems in adult life (aortic valve stenosis, SBE). Floppy mitral valve occurs in 5%.
Functional classification.
- **Acyanotic** = Obstruction: 10% pulmonary stenosis, 7% aortic stenosis, 7% coarctation of the aorta.
- **Potentially cyanotic** = hole with left to right shunt, cyanosis develops when Eisenmenger's reaction leads to a right to left shunt: 25% VSD, 12% patent ductus arteriosus, 10% atrial septal defects.
- **Cyanotic** = hole with right to left shunt: 7% tetralogy of Fallot, 7% transposition of the great vessels.

Prognosis. 40% are mild, 20% survive after emergency surgery as neonates, 20% survive after elective surgery in infancy or childhood, 20% die. All patients who have had surgery require cardiological follow-up for life.

PULMONARY STENOSIS
At risk: Rubella syndrome.
Pathology. Usually fusion or malformation of the valve. Sometimes subvalve stenosis, supravalve stenosis or pulmonary branch artery stenosis. Severe stenosis is associated with hypoplasia of the right ventricle.
Clinically.
- Mild stenosis remains asymptomatic, the systolic murmur is quiet and the pulmonary component of the second heart sound is delayed.
- Moderate stenosis is often detected in an asymptomatic child as a loud ejection systolic murmur in the pulmonary area with a single second heart sound. Without surgical correction heart failure often develops. Angina and syncope on exertion.
- Severe stenosis presents in the neonatal period with heart failure and cyanosis (despite classification as an acyanotic lesion).

Investigation. CxR may show an enlarged right ventricle and atrium. Echocardiogram is diagnostic. Cardiac catheterisation determines treatment.
Treatment and prognosis.
- Mild stenosis (30 mmHg systolic pressure gradient across the stenosis) - no treatment. Normal life expectancy and good health.

- Moderate stenosis (30-60 mmHg gradient) - observe. 5% operative mortality with subsequent good health for survivors.
- Severe stenosis (>60 mmHg gradient) - needs balloon angioplasty or open valvotomy. 30-80% operative mortality.

AORTIC STENOSIS

Pathology. 83% valvular stenosis, 9% subvalvar stenosis, 8% supravalvar stenosis.

Clinically.
- Usually found as an asymptomatic murmur.
- Sometimes presents with breathlessness, syncope, angina or sudden death on exertion. Weak pulse. Harsh ejection systolic murmur in the aortic area radiating to the neck. Reversed splitting of the second heart sound.
- Occasionally presents with heart failure in infancy.

Investigation. CxR may show left heart enlargement and post-stenotic dilatation. Echocardiogram is diagnostic. Cardiac catheterisation determines treatment.

Treatment. Mild stenosis (30 mmHg systolic pressure gradient across the stenosis) - no treatment except antibiotic prophylaxis for surgery (high risk of SBE). Moderate stenosis (30-60 mmHg gradient) - observe. Severe stenosis (>60 mmHg gradient) - needs balloon angioplasty or open valvotomy. Repeat valvotomy is often needed. Valve replacement in adult life for regurgitation or recurrent stenosis.

Prognosis. Heart failure in infancy - 50% operative mortality. After infancy - 5% operative mortality.

COARCTATION OF THE AORTA

Commonly 'Adult type' coarctation. Males > females. A discrete stenosis distal to the junction with the ductus arteriosus (ligamentum arteriosum). Collaterals develop in the chest wall between the subclavian arteries and the aorta below the stenosis (rib notching on CxR). Usually an incidental finding (weak or delayed femoral pulses, right arm hypertension, soft mid or late systolic murmur in the pulmonic area with radiation to the back, bruit of collaterals). May present in early adult life with complications (intracranial haemorrhage, heart failure, aortic rupture, aortitis). 50% have a bicuspid aortic valve that is prone to stenosis and SBE. Echocardiography is diagnostic but aortography is needed to define the lesion before surgery. Hypertension persists if surgical repair (end-to-end anastomosis) is delayed to late childhood.

Less commonly 'Infantile type' coarctation. Commonest cause of neonatal heart failure. A tubular stenosis proximal to the junction with the ductus arteriosus (DA). The DA usually remains patent carrying blood from the pulmonary trunk to the aorta below the stenosis. Delay or weakness of the femoral pulses is difficult to detect unless the DA closes. Left heart abnormalities are common (VSD, aortic stenosis, left heart hypoplasia). Prostaglandin E infusion keeps the DA open and the neonate alive until surgery (subclavian flap aortoplasty). Operative mortality in neonates is 5% for isolated coarctation, and 25% with associated left heart abnormalities. Operative mortality is 1% for asymptomatic infants (60% mortality without surgery). Definitive surgery (end-to-end anastomosis) in early childhood has an operative mortality of 1%.

EISENMENGER SYNDROME
Pathophysiology. If a congenital abnormality allows blood to flow from the left side of the heart to the right, the pulmonary arteries are exposed to increased flows and increased pressures. The pulmonary vascular resistance increases as the arterioles hypertrophy. Once pulmonary arterial pressure exceeds systemic arterial pressure desaturated blood is shunted from the right side of the heart to the left and the patient becomes cyanosed = Eisenmenger syndrome. This reversal develops rapidly with a high pressure shunt (VSD) and slowly with a low pressure shunt (ASD).
Symptoms. Fatigue, breathlessness, chest pain and syncope on exertion. Haemoptysis. Sudden death.
Signs. Of pulmonary hypertension + small volume pulse, low blood pressure, peripheral cyanosis (central cyanosis and clubbing are uncommon). There may be an early diastolic murmur of pulmonary regurgitation or a systolic murmur of tricuspid regurgitation. Pulmonary infarction (thrombosis in situ) is common from late adolescence. Pregnancy, anaesthesia and surgery can be fatal because of the restricted cardiac output.
Investigations. CxR and echocardiogram confirm right ventricular hypertrophy.
Treatment. Inoperable once established.

VENTRICULAR SEPTAL DEFECT (VSD)
Pathology. VSDs are usually single. As the pulmonary artery resistance falls following birth the VSD allows blood to flow from the left ventricle to the lower pressure right ventricle. This results in right heart strain and pulmonary hypertension.

Clinically. Harsh praecordial pan-systolic murmur.
* Some children develop right heart failure with feeding difficulties, failure to thrive and chest infections.
* Some develop Eisenmenger syndrome in adolescence or early adult life.
* Usually asymptomatic.

Investigations. ECG may suggest hypertrophy and strain of one or both sides of the heart. CxR may show cardiomegaly. Cardiac catheterisation: pulmonary artery pressure guides treatment.

Treatment. Antibiotic prophylaxis for surgery. Digoxin and diuretics usually control heart failure in infants. Children who remain symptomatic on drugs or have a rising pulmonary artery pressure should have a patch closure of the VSD before age 2. Children with large shunts have elective patch closure after age 3 to prevent heart failure or Eisenmenger syndrome developing.

Prognosis. 60% of VSDs close by age 3 years. Large VSDs or those associated with other cardiac defects rarely close. 10% operative mortality in infancy. 2% operative mortality after infancy. Life expectancy following surgery is nearly normal.

PATENT DUCTUS ARTERIOSUS (PDA)

Pathophysiology. In utero the lungs are collapsed and the pulmonary vascular resistance is very high. Blood is diverted from the left pulmonary artery through the ductus arteriosus into the aorta. At delivery the lungs expand and the pulmonary vascular resistance falls. The ductus arteriosus closes functionally within a few days of birth but anatomical closure takes 3-6 months. In premature babies the ductus arteriosus remains patent much longer. A PDA allows a left to right shunt and pulmonary hypertension. Eisenmenger's syndrome develops in early adult life (toes cyanosed before hands).

Clinically. Commonest cause of heart failure in premature neonates. A common cause of heart failure in the second month after delivery. Strong pulses, continuous murmur in the pulmonary area.

Investigation. Echocardiography is diagnostic.

Treatment. Infants with heart failure need diuretics prior to ligation of the PDA. Intravenous indomethacin will induce duct closure in 70% of symptomatic preterm infants. Elective ligation of the duct at six months in all others.

Prognosis. Average age at death if untreated is 36 years (SBE, LVF Eisenmenger syndrome). Operative mortality in infancy is 1% and life expectancy is then normal.

ATRIAL SEPTAL DEFECT (ASD)

Incidence. Girls (66%).

Pathophysiology.

- 70% ostium secundum ASD. The defect is in or around the septum secundum.
- 30% ostium primum ASD. A defect at the junction of the atrial septum and ventricular septum. There is usually a cleft in the mitral valve leaflet which is attached to the other side of the septum (mitral regurgitation). Sometimes there is a shunt from the left ventricle to the right atrium. Pulmonary hypertension develops in the 10% with bigger shunts.

Clinically.

- Ostium secundum ASD is usually asymptomatic in childhood, but 75% have atrial fibrillation and heart failure by age 50.
- Ostium primum ASD causes heart failure earlier in life, sometimes in infancy but invariably by age 30. Pulse normal unless arrhythmia. Fixed splitting of the second heart sound. Pulmonary ejection systolic murmur and mid-diastolic tricuspid murmur reflect increased flow. Mitral regurgitation. Cyanosis is uncommon.

Investigation. CxR may show cardiomegaly. ECG shows right axis deviation with secundum ASD and left axis deviation with primum ASD. Echocardiography is diagnostic, but cardiac catheterisation determines the need for surgery.

Treatment. Heart failure in infancy due to a large ASD may respond to digoxin and diuretics or require urgent patch closure (operative mortality 10%). A large asymptomatic ASD should be closed after age 2 (operative mortality 2%). Adults with pulmonary hypertension and heart failure have a 20% operative mortality for closure of their ASD. A small ASD can be left.

Prognosis. Normal life expectancy after surgical closure of a secundum ASD but atrial fibrillation can develop years later. Survival after closure of a primum defect depends on whether mitral valve disease develops.

TETRALOGY OF FALLOT

Incidence. Children with an affected parent have a 10% incidence of congenital heart disease.

Pathology. The bulbus cordis is divided into pulmonary trunk and aorta by a septum that grows down to fuse with the interventricular septum. If the septum deviates to the right:

The ventricular septum is incomplete (VSD).

The right ventricle outflow tract is narrowed (infundibular pulmonary stenosis).

- The aortic root opens partly into the right ventricle (over-riding aorta).
- Compensatory right ventricle hypertrophy.

Clinically. Pink at birth. Cyanosis develops in late infancy, as the pulmonary stenosis worsens. Episodes of breathlessness, palpitations, syncope and convulsions. Squatting after exertion. Failure to thrive. Normal pulse and JVP until failure develops. Mild cyanosis. Clubbing. Harsh pulmonary ejection systolic murmur and single S_2.

Complications. Heart failure (unusual before adult life). Stroke (cerebral thrombosis due to polycythaemia). Cerebral abscess and SBE. Arrhythmia.

Investigations. Polycythaemia. ECG shows right atrial and ventricular hypertrophy. CxR heart size normal, pulmonary oligaemia.

Treatment.
- General care: maintain hydration (reduces risk of stroke), iron supplements (prevent anaemia), oral propranolol (prevent cyanotic attacks).
- Cyanotic attacks: knee-chest position, oxygen, i.v. propranolol and sodium bicarbonate.
- Surgery. Aged < 6 months with severe cyanosis - subclavian to pulmonary artery shunt (hospital mortality <3%). Older than 6 months - definitive repair (hospital mortality <10%).

Prognosis. Without surgery 30% die in infancy and 75% die by age 10. 95% of those who survive definitive surgery live more than 8 years.

TRANSPOSITION OF THE GREAT ARTERIES

Pathophysiology. The aorta arises from the right ventricle and the pulmonary artery arises from the left ventricle. After placental separation survival is only possible if a shunt allows mixing between the two circulations (PDA, ASD, VSD). The bigger the shunt the better.

Clinically. Usually present in the first week with severe cyanosis, acidosis and cardiac failure.

Investigation. Echocardiogram is diagnostic but cardiac catheterisation is needed to define the anatomy.

Treatment. Prostaglandin E infusion to keep the ductus arteriosus open. Balloon atrial septostomy. Digoxin and diuretics for heart failure. Definitive surgery in early infancy (hospital mortality 10-30% depending on the severity of the associated defects).

Prognosis. Untreated 95% die in infancy. 95% 5-year survival after definitive surgery.

INFECTIVE ENDOCARDITIS

Incidence. Rare in infancy. Commoner with age.

Risk factors.
Usually:
- Most have classical CHD (VSD, aortic stenosis, tetralogy of Fallot, transposition of the great vessels).
- Intra-cardiac prostheses (valves > patches > pacemaker electrodes).
Sometimes:
- Acquired valve disease (rheumatic mitral valve).
- Bicuspid aortic valve, mitral valve prolapse.
- HOCM.
- Intravascular cannulae (shunts for hydrocephalus, feeding lines).
Previous infective endocarditis is also a risk factor.
Route of infection. Usually unknown. 25% follow a surgical (including dental) procedure. Sometimes sepsis (abscesses).
Infecting organism.
- 50% Streptococcus viridans (tends to cause subacute endocarditis).
- 30% Staphylococcus aureus (tends to cause acute endocarditis).
- 10% others (Candida, Staphylococcus albus).
- 10% no organism identified.
Pathology.
- Acute endocarditis rapidly destroys valves.
- Subacute endocarditis causes gradual destruction and vegetations accumulate (platelets, fibrin, organisms and phagocytes). Immune complexes cause petechiae and glomerulonephritis.
Clinically.
- **Acute endocarditis** causes severe toxicity, fever and rapidly progressive heart failure.
- **Subacute endocarditis** causes fever, malaise, weight loss, splenomegaly and petechiae. A murmur may appear or change. Rarely Osler nodes, splinter haemorrhages and emboli.
Investigations. Venous blood cultures are positive in 90% of patients. Serology for Chlamydia and Coxiella. Anaemia and raised ESR. Echocardiogram shows vegetations.
Treatment.
- Antibiotic prophylaxis for surgery and dental care.
- Acute or subacute endocarditis: antibiotics by i.v. bolus for 4-6 weeks.
- Surgery for progressive heart failure and recurrent emboli.
After clinical cure monitor fever (home charting). Repeat ESR, blood cultures and echocardiogram for signs of recurrence.
Prognosis. Invariably fatal if untreated. 20% mortality if treated.

ARRHYTHMIAS

Incidence. Rare in childhood.
Classification.

- **Paroxsymal supraventricular tachycardia.** Commonest childhood arrhythmia. 15% have an ectopic atrial pacemaker. 85% have an abnormal conduction pathway between the atrium and ventricles that allows a re-entry circuit (e.g. Woolf-Parkinson-White syndrome). Occasionally prolonged attacks cause heart failure, syncope or angina. Increasing vagal tone by the valsalva manoeuvre or carotid sinus massage often stops the tachycardia. Verapamil or amiodarone for resistant cases. Some need cardiac surgery to ablate a re-entry pathway.
- **Atrial fibrillation, atrial flutter, ventricular tachycardias** are rare except with cardiomyopathy or after cardiac surgery.
- **First-degree heart block** (slow AV node conduction - prolonged PR interval) in atrial septal defect, Ebstein's anomaly, myocarditis, digoxin therapy.
- **Second-degree heart block** (some P waves not conducted): congenital heart disease, myocarditis.
- **Third-degree heart block** (atria and ventricles disassociated): congenital heart disease and post-cardiac surgery. Ventricular rate 60 in infancy falling to 40 per minute in adolescence. Pacemaker for syncope.

14. HAEMATOLOGY

NORMAL VALUES

Haemoglobin (Hb).
- Fetus at term. Normal Hb = 17 g/dl (range 14–22). 50% is fetal Hb (HbF) which has a higher oxygen affinity suited to the relative hypoxia intra-utero.
- Infant. On delivery erythropoesis is suppressed because in conditions of relative hyperoxia HbF makes more oxygen available to the tissues than adult haemoglobin (HbA). As fetal red cells die they are not replaced. Erythropoetin secretion and erythropoesis restart at age 2–3 months when mean Hb = 10 g/dl of which 5% is HbF. By age 1 the mean Hb = 12 g/dl (HbF = 0).
- Age 12. Hb = 12. Adult values are reached at puberty.

White blood count varies little from infancy to adult life, but lymphocytes are commoner than neutrophils before age 5 falling to adult levels thereafter.

Platelet count varies little with age.

ANAEMIA

Aetiology.
1. Usually iron deficiency.
2. Sometimes:
   - Dilutional (growth exceeds erythropoesis in premature babies)
   - Folate deficiency.
3. Occasionally:
   - Globin synthesis defects (thalassaemia).
   - Haem synthesis defects (sideroblastic anaemia).
   - Marrow suppression (uraemia, hypothyroidism, chronic infection, disseminated malignancy).
   - Marrow aplasia.

Clinically. Pale, irritable, easily tired, anorexic. Compensatory increase in cardiac output (tachycardia, systolic flow murmur, cardiomegaly). Extramedullary haemopoiesis (splenomegaly, distorted bones).

Investigation.
- Full blood count and film: no further investigation is needed if a typical iron deficiency picture is found (reticulocytes <1%, low serum iron, raised transferrin, low ferritin, normal ESR) *and* the history and examination suggest dietary iron deficiency.

- Occult blood loss: if faecal occult blood is positive do upper and lower gastrointestinal endoscopy, urine analysis for blood (if positive do IVP).
- Malabsorption: microscopy and culture of faeces, serum B12, red cell folate.
- Haemolysis - see below.
- Occult infection: MSU for microscopy and culture, CxR.
- Metabolic disorder: creatinine, thyroxine, bilirubin.
- Marrow biopsy.

IRON DEFICIENCY ANAEMIA
Incidence. Common during rapid growth (infancy > adolescence). 30% of children aged 6-24 months. 60% in social class V. Premature infants are especially vulnerable because of more rapid growth and smaller iron stores. A GP will treat 3-6 children per year.
Aetiology.
- Usually dietary insufficiency: breast milk contains little iron, formula milk contains but insufficient iron supplements once iron stores have been used up (6 months old), vegans absorb little iron from egg and vegetables.
- Sometimes: malabsorption (coeliac) or chronic blood loss (gastrointestinal, urinary, menstruation).
Differential diagnosis of microcytic anaemia.
- Iron deficiency.
- Other defects of haem synthesis (sideroblastic anaemias, lead poisoning)
- Globin synthesis defects (thalassaemia).
Treatment.
- Prophylaxis: iron supplements to infants at risk, dietary advice.
- Established anaemia: oral iron (reticulosis starts after a 10-day lag then Hb increases by 1 g/dl every 10 days).
- Transfuse if anaemia is causing severe heart failure or a co-existing condition is suppressing haemopoesis.

MEGALOBLASTIC ANAEMIA
Incidence. Usually dietary folate deficiency with increased requirements (prematurity, infection, chronic haemolysis) or malabsorption (coeliac). B12 deficiency is very rare in childhood.
Pathology. Folate and B12 are essential for DNA synthesis. In folate or B12 deficiency the RBCs are big (macrocytes) because the pronormoblast divides fewer times before haemoglobinisation switches off cell division. Death of red cell precursors (ineffective erythropoiesis).Affects other rapidly dividing cells: marrow, epithelium (gut, respiratory, urogenital), gonads, osteoblasts.

Clinically.
- Anaemia.
- Mild jaundice (ineffective erythropoiesis), splenomegaly.
- Neutropenia: infections.
- Thrombocytopenia: bleeding.
- Diarrhoea.
- Neuropathy (B12 deficiency).

Treatment. Folic acid 5 mg daily.

SIDEROBLASTIC ANAEMIA
Pathology. Anaemia with severe iron loading of red cell precursors and ineffective erythropoiesis. Widespread haemosiderosis.

Incidence. Rare.

Aetiology. Congenital (usually X-linked), Acquired (cytotoxics).

Investigation. Mild to moderate anaemia (mixed normochromic and hypochromic RBCs). Marrow contains 'ring sideroblasts' (RBC precursors with a ring of iron granules around the nucleus).

Investigation. Normal Hb electrophoresis excludes thalassaemia.

Treatment. Pyridoxine sometimes helps.

APLASTIC ANAEMIA
Pathology. A reduced number of erythroblasts in the bone marrow. Myeloblasts and megakaryocytes are usually also reduced.

Incidence. Very rare.
- 30%   congenital (often familial).
- 70%   acquired: idiopathic, chloramphenicol, cytotoxics, radio-therapy.

Clinically. Anaemia, infection, bleeding. No hepatosplenomegaly or generalised lymphadenopathy.

Differential diagnosis of pancytopenia.
- Aplastic anaemia: marrow contains few precursor cells.
- Acute leukaemia: marrow packed with blast cells.
- Idiopathic thrombocytopenic purpura (ITP): marrow normal except for numerous megakaryocytes.

Investigation: anaemia, neutropenia, thrombocytopenia. ESR is very high. Blood film: mainly normal red cells, low reticulocyte count (<1%), no abnormal blast cells. Bone marrow: fat cells but very few precursor cells.

Treatment. General treatment appropriate for immuno-incompetent patients. Corticosteroids and androgens are of little or no benefit. Bone marrow transplantation (BMT) for severe disease.

Prognosis. 60% long term survival after BMT (30% without).

HAEMOLYTIC ANAEMIA

Pathology. Shortened RBC survival (normal = 120 days). RBCs may be destroyed in the circulation (intra-vascular haemolysis) or in the reticulo-endothelial system (extra-vascular haemolysis). The consequences of haemolysis are:

1. Increased RBC production:
   • Erythroid hyperplasia: the erythroid marrow spreads down the long bones.
   • Extramedullary haemopoiesis: in congenital haemolysis blood is made in the liver, spleen and lymph nodes.
   • Reticulocytosis.
2. Intravascular haemolysis releases Hb.
   • Hb–haptoglobin complexes are taken up by the reticulo-endothelial system (RES).
   • Once the haptoglobin is exhausted, the Hb is degraded to haem in the circulation and binds to haemopexin.
   • Once the haemopexin is saturated the haem binds to albumin (methaemalbumin).
   • Severe haemolysis results in free Hb which is filtered by the kidneys and appears in the urine as haemosiderin.
   • Massive haemolysis results in free haemoglobin in the urine.
3. Unconjugated bilirubin released from Hb appears as increased urinary and fecal urobilinogen (dark urine and stools).

Aetiology.
• Immune disorders.
• Inherited red cell defects (spherocytosis, G6PDH deficiency, haemoglobinopathies).
• Micro-angiopathic haemolytic anaemia (haemolytic uraemic syndrome).
• Secondary hypersplenism.
• Infections (septicaemia, malaria).

Investigation.
• **Is there haemolysis?** Reticulocytosis (>20%), polychromatic macrocytosis, raised serum unconjugated bilirubin.
• **Is the haemolysis intravascular?** reduced haptoglobin, methaemalbumin present, haemoglobinuria (massive haemolysis) or haemosiderin in the urine (chronic haemolysis).
• **Where in the RES are red cells being destroyed?** Radioactive chromium labelled red cell studies.
• **What is causing the haemolysis?** G6PDH, osmotic fragility and sugar test, Coombs test, sickle test, Hb electrophoresis.

Immune haemolytic anaemia
Aetiology.
* Isoimmune: Abs against Rhesus and ABO antigens are transferred from mother to fetus. See 'Jaundice'.
* Autoimmune: usually idiopathic. Sometimes Abs raised against an infection or drug cross react with red cell antigens. Sometimes Abs raised against drugs lyse red cells to which the drug is bound. Anti-RBC Abs occur in lymphoma, leukaemia and SLE.

Clinically.
* **Warm haemolysis**. Red cells with attached IgG are cleared by splenic macrophages (extravascular haemolysis). Anaemia. Splenomegaly.
* **Cold haemolysis**. RBCs with IgM attached are cleared by reticulo-endothelial cells in the liver (extravascular haemolysis), agglutinated in the cold (Raynaud's syndrome), and lysed by complement when cold (acute intravascular haemolysis causes haemoglobinuria, abdominal pain, jaundice). Often follows mycoplasma or viral infections.

Investigations. Direct Coomb's positive for IgM and Indirect Coomb's test positive for IgG.

Treatment and prognosis. Transfusion.
* Warm haemolysis often remits spontaneously. Helped by prednisolone, chlorambucil and splenectomy.
* Cold haemolysis is helped by keeping warm and plasma exchange. Post–infective cases are usually transient and seldom recur. Severe intravascular haemolysis can cause acute renal failure and aplastic crises.

Hereditary spherocytosis
Incidence. 3/1,000. Boys = girls. Caucasian. Autosomal dominant (25% are new mutations).

Pathogenesis. Membrane is too permeable to sodium. Intracellular fluid accumulation makes the cell spherical so it is trapped and destroyed in the spleen.

Clinically. Mild to moderate anaemia. Infections can precipitate severe haemolytic or aplastic anaemia. Gallstones. Splenomegaly. Leg ulcers.

Investigations. Spherocytes on blood film, but these can occur with other causes of haemolysis. Positive osmotic fragility test. Autohaemolysis partially reversed by glucose.

Treatment. Folic acid supplements. Transfusions for haemolytic or aplastic crises. Splenectomy largely prevents haemolysis although spherocytosis persists.

Glucose 6-phosphate dehydrogenase deficiency

Incidence. X-linked recessive. Affects 100 million people.

Pathology. G6PDH is the first enzyme in the pentose phosphate pathway which protects red cells from oxidation. If G6PDH is deficient red cells are vulnerable to intravascular haemolysis.

Clinically. A variety of syndromes:

- **Favism.** Common in the Mediterranean countries, Middle East, and Far East. Acute intravascular haemolysis 6-24 hours after eating broad beans, or oxidant drugs (anti-malarials, sulphonamides, NSAIDs) and during viral infections or acidosis. Neonatal jaundice. Improves with age.
- **Primaquine sensitivity.** Common in West Africa and Thailand. Intravascular haemolysis a few days after starting primaquine. Haemolysis stops if primaquine is continued because new red cells contain more G6PDH. Neonatal jaundice.
- **Congenital extravascular haemolysis.** Rare and sporadic.

Investigations. Blood film: distorted red cells containing clumps of oxidised Hb (Heinz bodies). Red cell G6PDH activity low.

Treatment. Avoid precipitants. Prognosis is good.

Sickle cell anaemia

Incidence. 10% of black people carry the gene for HbS. Homo-zygotes have sickle cell anaemia. Heterozygotes have sickle cell trait.

Pathology. RBCs containing HbS tend to sickle and form stacks when hypoxic. Sickled cells are cleared by the spleen and may block vessels. Autosplenectomy by repeated infarcts, predisposes to sepsis.

Clinically. Anaemia. Painful venocclusive crises. Frequent bacterial infections causing haemolytic, aplastic and sequestration crises. Gallstones. Swollen tender fingers (dactylitis). Salmonella arthritis and osteomyelitis. Aseptic necrosis of the femoral head. Microvascular occlusion eventually causes chronic hepatic and renal failure.

Treatment.

- Folic acid supplements.
- Prevent sickle crises: avoid dehydration, acidosis and hypoxia (air travel).
- Prevention of sepsis: prophylactic penicillin throughout childhood and additional antibiotics for suspected sepsis. Polyvalent pneumococcal vaccine at age 2 years.
- Sickle crisis: narcotic analgesics, oxygen, intravenous fluids, whole blood transfusion.

Prognosis. Homozygotes rarely live beyond middle age. Heterozygotes only sickle under extreme anoxia.

Thalassaemia
Incidence. Autosomal recessive. Up to 30% are heterozygous in countries around the Mediteranean, India and the Far East. Beta-thalassaemia is more common than alpha–thalassaemia.
Pathology. Haemoglobin is made up of two pairs of globulin chains. Each pair carries one haem group.

HbA	= 2 alpha-chains + 2 beta-chains.
HbA2	= 2 alpha + 2 delta.
HbF	= 2 alpha + 2 gamma.
Embryonic Hb	= 2 epsilon + 2 gamma.

Each chromosome-16 carries genes for 2 alpha-chains. Each chromosome-11 carries genes for 2 gamma, 1 beta, 1 delta and 1 epsilon chain. In thalassaemia some of these genes are absent or suppressed.

Alpha-thalassaemia
No alpha-chains = Hydrops fetalis. The fetal Hb largely consists of tetramers of gamma-chains (haemoglobin Bart's). The fetus usually dies in the third trimester as embryonic Hb levels decline. Severe anaemia, generalised oedema, massive hepatosplenomegaly. The mother often develops eclamptic toxaemia.
Alpha-chains 25% of normal = Haemoglobin H disease. Only 1 of the 4 alpha-chain genes is expressed. HbH is a tetramer of beta-chains. Microcytic anaemia. Hb = 9 g/dl = 40% HbH + 57% HbA + 3% HbA2. HbH does not precipitate in erythroid cells (erythropoiesis is relatively normal so marrow hyperplasia is mild). HbH precipitates in erythrocytes which are cleared by the spleen. Episodes of severe haemolysis caused by pregnancy, infections and oxidant drugs (sulphonamides). Most live to adult life.
Alpha-chains 50% of normal = alpha-thal trait. Mild microcytic anaemia. Normal Hb electrophoresis.
Alpha-chains 75% of normal = silent carrier. Mild microcytosis but no anaemia and normal Hb electrophoresis.

Beta-thalassaemia.
No beta-chains = Thalassaemia major. Hypochromic, microcytic anaemia with Hb = 2-8 g/dl = 97% HbF + 3% HbA2. Marked erythroid hyperplasia of the marrow but many RBC precursors are destroyed by precipitated alpha-chains (ineffective erythropoiesis) so there is only a mild reticulocytosis. Pale infant who fails to thrive and suffers recurrent infections.
• If adequately transfused (monthly) development is normal and splenomegaly minimal. However, iron overload develops by age 10 with failure of the

adolescent growth spurt, diabetes, hypoparathyroidism, adrenal insufficiency, and liver failure. Die with cardiac failure or sudden death aged 15 to 25. Intensive chelation therapy (desferrioxamine and ascorbic acid) may improve prognosis. Splenectomy for hypersplenism. Bone marrow transplantation is of unproven benefit.
- If inadequately transfused growth is slow, marrow expands the skull vault, long bones suffer recurrent fractures, there is massive splenomegaly, and recurrent infections. The few who survive to puberty develop iron overload.
- Untransfused all die in infancy.

Some beta-chains = Thalassaemia intermedia. A variety of gene defects. Moderate anaemia. Symptoms vary from none to almost as bad as thalassaemia major. Seldom transfusion dependent.

50% of normal beta-chains = Thalassaemia minor. Heterozygote. Hb=11 g/dl. 90% HbA + 5% HbA2 (high) + 5% HbF (high). Mild reticulocytosis. Asymptomatic. Mild splenomegaly in 30%. At risk for gallstones and folate deficiency in pregnancy.

BRUISING AND BLEEDING

Aetiology.
Neonate:
- Trauma: birth trauma.
- Infection: congenital rubella, syphilis, toxoplasmosis, septicaemia.
- Thrombocytopenia: isoantibodies (ABO incompatibility), auto-antibodies (SLE), drugs, cavernous haemangioma.

At any age the common causes are:
- Trauma: accidental, non-accidental, coughing.
- Vasculitis: Henoch-Schönlein purpura (HSP).
- Defective platelet function: aspirin and NSAIDs.
- Thrombocytopenia: idiopathic thrombocytopenic purpura (ITP).
- Infection: septicaemia.

At any age the uncommon causes are:
- Thrombocytopenia: leukaemia, lymphoma, hypersplenism, disseminated intravascular coagulation (DIC).
- Defective platelet function: congenital, uraemia.
- Clotting deficiencies: haemophilia, warfarin, vitamin K deficiency, liver disease.
- Abnormal blood vessels: vasculitis (haemolytic uraemic syndrome, SLE), scurvy, Cushing's syndrome, collagen disorders.

Investigation. FBC and film. Clotting function and clotting factors. Bleeding time. Marrow aspirate.

HENOCH-SCHONLEIN PURPURA
Incidence. Boys > girls. Age 5.
Pathology. Vasculitis.
Clinically. Urticaria then purpura on extensor surfaces of the lower limbs, buttocks. Arthritis. Abdominal pain and intestinal bleeding. Nephritis with haematuria (40%).
Investigations. All normal.
Prognosis. 80% spontaneous resolution. 20% chronic glomerulonephritis and renal failure. 40% have a recurrence.

IDIOPATHIC THROMBOCYTOPAENIC PURPURA
Incidence. Age 3-7 years. Boys = girls.
Pathology. Antibodies against platelets and megakaryocytes.
Clinically. Sudden onset of purpura may be preceded by a recognised viral infection. No splenomegaly.
Investigations. Low platelets. Normal Hb and WBC. Occasional atypical lymphocyte. Marrow biopsy to exclude leukaemia.
Treatment. Prednisolone until platelet count normal. Chronic ITP is treated by splenectomy and azathioprine.
Prognosis. 80% recover within a few weeks, 20% develop chronic ITP.

HAEMOPHILIA
Incidence. X-linked recessive. Prevalence in UK is 8,000 (50% mild). A GP will see one new case every 600 years.
Pathology. Non-functional Factor VIII is made in normal amounts.

% normal function of Factor VIII	Clinical effect
1-5	Spontaneous bruising and haemarthroses.
5-25	Gross bleeding after minor injuries.
25-50	Slight delay in clotting.
50-100	Normal.

Treatment. Factor VIII cryoprecipitate.
Prognosis. Progressive joint destruction by recurrent haemarthroses if there is less than 25% of the normal Factor VIII function. Hepatitis and HIV infection from factor VIII concentrates.

IMMUNE DEFICIENCY

- Congenital: cyclic neutropenia, various rare immune deficiency syndromes.
- Acquired: HIV infection, immunosuppressive therapy (cortico-steroids, radiotherapy, cytotoxics), leukaemia, lymphoma, aplastic anaemia, hypersplenism

ACQUIRED IMMUNE DEFICIENCY SYNDROME (AIDS)

Incidence. Uncommon but increasing.

Pathology. 60% of HIV infected mothers will infect their fetus infection by transplacental transmission. T-helper cells (T4) are infected by the Human Immune Deficiency Virus (HIV) and lysed when the virus has replicated. Recurrent infections (pyogenic, tuberculosis, herpes viruses, Candida, Pneumocystis carinii pneumonia, Toxoplasma gondii meningitis). Lymphoma. Dementia. Myopathy. Arthritis. Kaposi's sarcoma is very rare.

Clinically. Lymphadenopathy, sweats, weight loss. Recurrent infections from age 2.

Investigation. T-helper cell count. Pancytopenia. Elevated serum immunoglobulins.

Treatment. Offer ante-natal screening to high risk groups and offer termination of pregnancy to HIV infected mothers. Avoid infections. Antibiotics, antifungals and anti-viral agents as indicated. Zidovudine inhibits the replication of HIV but frequently causes anaemia.

Prognosis. Usually survive less than 2 years from onset of illness.

LYMPHADENOPATHY

- Infection (local, systemic).
- Immune deficiency.
- Collagen disorders: JCA.
- Neoplasia: leukaemia, lymphoma.
- Granulomatous diseases: sarcoidosis.

LEUKAEMIA

Incidence. 3.5/100,000 children each year. Age 0-5 years. A GP would see one new case every 200 years. At risk: identical twin with leukaemia, Down's syndrome, Fanconi's aplastic anaemia.

- 85% Acute Lymphoblastic Leukaemia (ALL). Age 3-5.
- 14% Acute Myeloblastic Leukaemia (AML). Neonates.
- 1% Chronic Myeloid Leukaemia (CML).

Clinically. Sudden or insidious onset:
* Malaise, weight loss, fever.
* Bone marrow suppression: anaemia (normochromic, normocytic), infection (neutropenia), bruising (low platelets).
* Infiltration: bone pain, hepatosplenomegaly (ALL>AML), lymphadenopathy (localised in AML, widespread in ALL), skin nodules, meninges (headache, vomiting and convulsions), painless testicular swelling (20% of boys).

Investigation. Leukaemic blast cells in the peripheral blood.

General management.
* Reverse barrier nursing when severely neutropenic.
* Systemic antibiotics if there is any suggestion of infection.
* Prophylactic oral antifungals during intensive cytotoxic therapy.
* Transfuse RBCs, WBCs and platelets as needed.
* Correct metabolic abnormalities during acute attacks and cytotoxic therapy: high fluid intake, allopurinol (hyperuricaemia), bicarbonate (acidosis).
* Psychological and social support for the patient and family.

Specific treatment of ALL.
* Remission in > 90% after 4 weeks of oral prednisolone and weekly i.v. vincristine. Intrathecal methotrexate, hydrocortisone and cytosine arabinoside reduces the meningeal recurrence rate from 80% to 10%.
* Maintenance cytotoxics for 3 years. No universally agreed regime.
* Relapse. Testicular infiltration is treated with radiotherapy, and meningeal infiltration with intrathecal methotrexate.
* Bone marrow transplantation during second remission.

Specific treatment of AML.
* Remission in > 80% of those given 3-weekly intravenous (doxorubicin, thioguanine and cytosine arabinoside) and intrathecal therapy until the marrow is clear.
* Maintenance cytotoxics for 3 years. No universally agreed regime.
* Bone marrow transplantation during first remission.

Prognosis. 5-year disease-free survival off maintenance therapy in 60% of cases of ALL and 30% of AML. Prognosis is better for boys with onset aged 1-8 years, no CNS involvement, no chromosomal abnormalities in the blast cells. Worse prognosis if circulating WBC > 20,000 at diagnosis.

LYMPHOMA

Malignant proliferations of lymphoid cells (lymphocytes and histiocytes). Arise in lymph nodes > spleen. Often spread to bone marrow but seldom flood the peripheral blood.

Hodgkin's lymphoma

Incidence. 35 children/ year in UK. Boys (3:1). Rare before puberty then increases in frequency with age.

Pathology. Characterised by multinucleated giant cells (Reed-Sternberg). The majority of malignant cells are small mononuclear cells. The degree of malignancy varies with the histology, increasing from lymphocytic predominance – nodular sclerosis – mixed cellularity – lymphocyte depletion.

Clinically. Present with discrete lymphadenopathy (cervical in 75%), weight loss, fever, anaemia. Splenomegaly in 50%. Other symptoms are due to enlarged nodes infiltrating or pressing on surrounding structures.

Investigation. Diagnosis by lymph node biopsy. Staging investigations as for adults except laparotomy is usually avoided.

Treatment. Involved field radiotherapy with six courses of MOPP (mustine, vincristine, procarbazine) for all stages. 90% cure rate.

Non-Hodgkin's lymphoma

Incidence. 7/million children. Incidence increases with age. 5% of childhood malignancies. A GP will see 1 new case every 5,000 years.

Pathology. Extra-nodal involvement is more common than in Hodgkin's disease and 2/3 are widely spread at diagnosis. Frequently converts to acute lymphoblastic leukaemia. Commoner in children with immune deficiencies.

Clinically. Matted lymph nodes, weight loss, fever, hepatosplenomegaly.

Treatment. Intensive chemotherapy and local radiotherapy cures 90% of localised disease and 35% of diffuse disease.

SPLENOMEGALY

Aetiology.
- Infection: infectious mononucleosis.
- Leukaemia, lymphoma.
- Secondary to extravascular haemolysis.
- Extra-medullary haematopoiesis.
- Collagen diseases: JCA, SLE.

Complications. Hypersplenism (destruction of RBCs and platelets in the spleen).

Management. Splenectomy is indicated for severe hypersplenism. The subsequent risk of Pneumococcal septicaemia is less if splenectomy is deferred until age 5 years, polyvalent pneumococcal vaccine is given before splenectomy, and prophylactic penicillin is given indefinitely (at least until age 12). There is an increased incidence of thrombosis after splenectomy.

15. ENDOCRINOLOGY AND METABOLISM

DIABETES MELLITUS
Incidence. 1/500 children. Usually insulin dependent. Onset usually 5-12 years old. Less strongly familial than adult onset diabetes, but 6% of siblings of a diabetic child will develop diabetes in childhood.
Aetiology.
Usually idiopathic (immune mediated pancreatic damage).
Occasionally:
- Infection (mumps, congenital rubella, coxsackie B).
- Pancreatic damage (cystic fibrosis, iron overload, surgery).
- Anti-insulins (growth hormone, corticosteroids).
- Congenital abnormality of the pancreas.
- Syndromes (Down's, Turner's, Klinefelter's).

Clinically. Usually present after a few days or weeks of tiredness, thirst, polyuria, bed wetting, skin infections. Occasionally present with abdominal pain, vomiting, and tachypnoea due to ketoacidosis. Complications in early adult life: retinopathy, microvascular disease, arteriopathy, glomerulonephritis and renal failure, neuropathy.

Diagnosis. Blood glucose >10 mmol/l confirms diagnosis.

Management. Educate the child to look after his own diabetes.
- Ketoacidosis is treated with i.v. fluids and i.v. insulin. Recurrent ketoacidosis suggests habitually poor glucose control + infection.
- Hypoglycaemia is treated with intramuscular glucagon followed by oral sugar when the child recovers sufficiently to drink.
- Insulin. A mixture of soluble and medium duration human insulin is given twice daily. Alternatively a long acting insulin is given once daily with soluble insulin before meals.
- Diet should be based on the food eaten by the rest of the family. Highly refined carbohydrates and fat should be discouraged. Fibre and unrefined carbohydrate should be encouraged.
- Self monitoring of blood glucose using a spring loaded lancet, test strip and reflectance meter.
- Annual or 6-monthly checks for complications and glucose control. The glycosylated haemoglobin level reflects the mean blood glucose over the preceding 3 months, and is the best predictor of complications.
- Exercise.
- Career choice.

Prognosis. Increased adult mortality due to renal failure (pyelonephritis > glomerulonephritis), and myocardial infarction.

HYPOGLYCAEMIA
Aetiology. Blood glucose < 2.2 mmol/l.
1. Usually a known diabetic after excessive insulin, unusual exercise, or a missed meal.
2. Sometimes reactive hypoglycaemia occurs 2-4 hours after a normal child eats a lot of refined carbohydrate.
3. Rarely.
     • Excessive production of insulin (islet cell hyperplasia, insulinoma).
     • Reduced anti-insulins (growth hormone or cortisol).
     • Liver fails to produce glucose during a fast (liver failure, galactosaemia, glycogen storage diseases).
Clinically. Hypoglycaemia causes hunger, irritability, blurred vision, and collapse. The adrenergic response to hypoglycaemia causes sweating, tremor, dilated pupils, and tachycardia.
Management. Give glucose. Refer for investigation unless known to be receiving medication for diabetes.

DIABETES INSIPIDUS (DI)
Aetiology. All causes are rare.
• Central DI = Antidiuretic hormone (ADH) deficiency. Usually idiopathic, sometimes due to pituitary damage.
• Nephrogenic DI = Kidney unresponsive to ADH.
Pathophysiology. ADH permits resorption of water from the collecting ducts. In DI too much water is lost.
Clinically. Polyuria, polydipsia, enuresis, dehydration, poor growth.
Investigation. Hypernatraemia but dilute urine.
Differential diagnosis of dilute urine. Compulsive water drinking; chronic renal failure; DI.
Treatment.
• Central DI: adequate intake of water and desmopressin nasal spray.
• Nephrogenic DI: thiazide diuretics.

CONGENITAL HYPOTHYROIDISM
Incidence. Girls (2:1). 1/4,000 infants in the UK (thyroid malformation or enzyme defect). In underdeveloped countries maternal iodine deficiency is the commonest cause.
Clinically. Sleepy baby. Prolonged neonatal jaundice. Hypotonia. Mild cases present in childhood and mimic acquired hypothyroidism.
Screening. In the UK blood taken on the 8th day after birth is tested for thyroid stimulating hormone (TSH). High levels sugest hypothyroidism.

Treatment. If L-thyroxine is not started before 3 months of age irreversible brain damage will occur.

ACQUIRED HYPOTHYROIDISM
Incidence. Uncommon. Uusually due to chronic autoimmune thyroiditis. Sometimes due to pituitary failure (low thyroid stimulating hormone (TSH)) or hypothalamic dysfunction (low thyrotrophin releasing hormone (TRH)).
Clinically. Growth failure. Goitre.
Investigation. Low thyroxine, high TSH and antibodies to thyroid microsomes suggest autoimmune thyroiditis.
Treatment. L-thyroxine results in normal height within 2 years.

HYPERTHYROIDISM
Graves' disease
Rare in childhood. Hyperactive child with weight loss, tachycardia, goitre and exophthalmos. Treatment with anti-thyroid drugs (carbimazole) > partial thyroidectomy.
Neonatal hypothyroidism
Rare. Due to transplacental transfer of antibody from a mother with Graves' disease. Lasts up to 3 months. Failure to thrive despite a huge appetite.

GOITRE
Incidence. 5% of teenagers. Girls (2:1).
Differential diagnosis of goitre.
- Simple goitre. A mild diffuse goitre often due to iodine deficiency. Occasionally due to dietary goitrogens including iodine. Normal thyroid function. Sporadic, common in adolescent girls.
- Autoimmune thyroiditis (Hashimoto's disease > Graves' disease).
- Thyroid cancer (rare in children).
- The thyroid fails to make or release thyroxine due to an enzyme defect. The TSH response causes diffuse goitre.

Investigation. Thyroid function and ultrasound.
Treatment. Thyroxine can reverse a simple goitre.

HYPOCALCAEMIA
Aetiology.
- Neonatal hypocalcaemia may occur if a neonate is given milk containing a lot of phosphate. Modern modified baby-milk powders are low in phosphate. Treat with calcium gluconate.

- Rickets = vitamin D deficiency: Inadequate cholecalciferol in the diet; malabsorption; lack of sunlight exposure; kidney disease affecting the activating hydroxylation of vitamin D. Responds to vitamin D analogues.
- Parathyroid destruction in childhood is due to autoimmune disease or surgery of the parathyroids. Treated with high dose Vitamin D analogues.
- Pseudohypoparathyroidism is due to a genetically determined end organ insensitivity to parathormone (PTH).

Clinically. Acute: tremor, tetany, convulsions. Chronic: rickets.

Differential diagnosis of tetany.
- Hypocalcaemia.
- Acidosis increases protein binding of calcium (hyperventilation).
- Hypomagnesaemia.

HYPERCALCAEMIA
- Vitamin D overdose.
- Idiopathic hypercalcaemia.
- Primary hyperparathyroidism.

Clinically. Vomiting, failure to thrive, constipation. Renal stones and renal impairment.

ADRENAL INSUFFICIENCY
Incidence. Usually due to withdrawal of corticosteroid therapy. Occasionally due to autoimmune Addison's disease.

Clinically. lethargy and weight loss.

Investigation. No cortisol response to synthetic ACTH.

Treatment. Oral prednisolone.

CONGENITAL ADRENAL HYPERPLASIA (CAH)
Incidence. Autosomal recessive. 1/5,000 live births.

Pathophysiology. Progesterone is hydroxylated at the 17th, 21st and 11th carbon atoms to make cortisol and aldosterone. The commonest defect (95%) is a deficiency of the 21-hydroxylase. This results in:
- A lack of cortisol. Increased ACTH often restores cortisol levels but causes adrenal hyperplasia.
- A lack of aldosterone. If severe this results in a salt-loosing crisis (hypokalaemia, acidosis, sodium loss and dehydration).
- Conversion of excess progesterone to androstenedione causes virilisation of a female and precocious puberty in a male. Early epiphyseal closure results in short stature.

Clinically. Ambiguous genitalia or a very sick baby.

Investigation. Plasma electrolytes should be measured as an emergency procedure on every baby with ambiguous genitalia. Elevated plasma 17-hydroxyprogesterone is diagnostic

Treatment. Correct acidosis and electrolyte abnormalities if present. Corticosteroid supplements. Plastic surgery for ambiguous genitals.

GROWTH DISORDERS

Failure to thrive

This term is applied to pre-school children. By definition 3% of children are abnormally small but only some of these are abnormal.

Aetiology.

1. Basically normal (small but not actually failing to thrive because growth velocity is normal).
   - Small child of small parents.
   - Low birth weight with failure to catch up.
   - Social or emotional deprivation.
   - Failure to catch up after prolonged systemic disease.
2. Defective intake is the commonest cause of failure to thrive.
   - Not offered enough milk or food. Especially breast-fed babies.
   - Difficulty swallowing: cerebral palsy.
   - Poor appetite due to disease, drugs or mental retardation.
   - Malabsorption: cystic fibrosis, coeliac disease.
3. Excessive loss of food: vomiting or diarrhoea.
4. Any severe, prolonged illness: heart disease, renal failure, JCA.
5. Genetic defects: chromosomal abnormalities; achondroplasia.
6. Endocrine abnormalities: deficiency of growth hormone (GH); hypothyroidism; diabetes mellitus; precocious puberty with premature closure of epiphyses.
7. Metabolic abnormalities.

Clinical assessment. Good social circumstances, good dietary intake, no symptoms and a normal growth velocity (height, weight and head circumference) for age suggests that the child is basically normal. Centile charts correcting for mid-parental height and premature delivery are often enlightening.

Investigations. If the clinical assessment was worrying a GP should refer the child to a paediatrician:
- Blood: FBC, ESR, glucose, electrolytes, pH, liver function, calcium, thyroid function.

- Urine: protein, blood and culture.
- X-ray hand for bone age. X-ray pituitary fossa.
- Other investigations as indicated: sweat test, jejunal biopsy, GH stimulation tests.

Treatment. Only 2,000 children are receiving GH injections, 1 for every 15 GPs.

Short stature

This term is applied to school age children. It can be due to all the causes of failure to thrive. It can also be due to delayed puberty.

Tall

Aetiology. By definition 3% of children are abnormally tall.
1. Basically normal
   - Tall child of tall parents.
   - Obesity (epiphyses tend to close at the mid-parental height).
2. Abnormal
   - Syndromic: Marfan's, Klinefelter's.
   - Endocrine: GH secreting adenoma, thyrotoxicosis, CAH.

Clinically. If the child is basically normal and growing along a centile line the child and parents can be reassured.

Investigation. X-ray hand for bone age. Thyroid function, 17-hydroxyprogesterone, GH suppression test. Karyotype.

Treatment. Growth can be halted by giving testosterone or oestrogen to close the epiphyses. Osteotomy to shorten the lower limbs.

SEXUAL MATURATION

The gonad differentiates into an ovary or a testis during the 6th week of embryonic life depending on the sex chromosomes. The gonad then determines the development of the internal sexual organs. The external genitalia differentiate into the male form if adequate androgens are present, otherwise they adopt the female form. At puberty the hypothalamus releases luteinizing hormone releasing hormone (LHRH). The pituitary then releases luteinizing hormone (LH) and follicle stimulating hormone (FSH) which stimulate gametogenesis. In girls breast development is followed by the growth spurt, redistribution of body fat, pubic hair and menstruation. In boys the growth of the testes is followed by the growth spurt, development of pubic hair, penile growth and deepening of the voice. Puberty ceases with epiphyseal closure.

Intersex
See 'Disorders of the genitals'.

Early sexual maturation
The development of sexual characteristics before age 8 in girls or 9.5 in boys.
- Precocious puberty implies early activation of the hypothalamic-pituitary-gonad axis. LH and FSH secretion cause gametogenesis.
- The isolated development of one (or two) secondary sexual characteristics such as pubic hair.
- Sexual precocity is the result of ectopic oestrogen secretion in girls and androgen secretion in boys.

Incidence. Rare. Commoner in girls (5:1).

Aetiology.

	Female	Male
• Idiopathic precocious puberty	75%	35%
• Hypothalamic or pituitary lesion	14%	43%
• Androgen secreting tumour or CAH	virilizes	22%
• Other, including HCG secreting tumour	11%	rare

Clinical assessment. Weight and height plotted on centile charts with previous data. Sexual characteristics. Visual fields.

Investigation. Blood levels of LH, FSH, oestradiol-17ß, testosterone, 17-hydroxyprogesterone. Hand X-ray for bone age. Pituitary fossa X-ray. Ultrasound or CT scan of hypothalamus, adrenals and ovaries.

Treatment. Idiopathic precocious puberty can be suppressed with danazol in girls and cyproterone acetate in boys.

Delayed puberty
Definition. No pubertal changes in a girl aged 13 or a boy aged 15.

Aetiology.
- Usually physiological (often familial).
- Commonly hypothalamic suppression by anorexia nervosa or systemic illness.
- Sometimes: chromosome abnormalities (Turner's, Klinefelter's).
- Occasionally: gonadotrophin releasing hormone deficiency; pituitary lesion (craniopharyngioma); pineal destruction, myxoedema, gonadal failure.

Clinical assessment. As for premature puberty. A pituitary lesion should be suspected when growth failure is marked.

Investigation. As for premature puberty + karyotype.

Treatment.
- LH or FSH deficiency. Puberty can be induced by injections of HCG. Then give testosterone (boys) or oestrogen (girls).
- Gonadal failure. Secondary sexual differentiation can be induced with oestrogen in girls and testosterone in boys. Treatment should be delayed until an acceptable height has been reached.

INBORN ERRORS OF METABOLISM
Pathology. Inherited, usually autosomal recessive, deficiencies in enzyme function. The ill effects are caused by:
- the lack of the normal end product.
- the accumulation of unused substrate.
- the formation of a toxic alternative metabolite.
- a combination of the above reasons.

Classification.
- Hyperlipidaemias.
- Aminoacid metabolism: phenylketonuria (1/10,000 live births); Homocystinuria (1/30,000).
- Sugar metabolism: galactosaemia (1/70,000), hereditary fructose intolerance.
- Glycogen storage diseases.
- Mucopolysaccharidoses (combined incidence 1/10,000): Hurler's syndrome, Hunter's syndrome.
- Lipid storage diseases: Tay-Sachs disease.
- Wilson's disease (copper accumulation).
- Others: urea cycle defects, porphyrias.

Clinically. Mental retardation and growth failure are common effects. Detailed descriptions of the commoner syndromes are given in the 'Textbook of Paediatrics' by Forfar and Arneil.

Management.
- Population screening (Guthrie test).
- Specific investigations of suspected cases.
- Diet and drug therapy can limit the damage caused by certain defects.
- Genetic counselling is discussed in the chapter on 'Genetic abnormalities'.

16. NEUROLOGY

THE AIMS OF PAEDIATRIC NEUROLOGY

- To diagnose abnormal development. Distinguish the static and progressive components of a disability. Identify specific causes of deterioration. Assess prognosis.
- To treat disease, minimise disability, and help the patient overcome handicap.
- To support the family of the patient.

HEADACHE

Incidence. 1 in 5 schoolchildren have at least 1 headache each year.
Aetiology.
- **Common acute:** any infection causing fever, localised infection of the head (sinusitis, otitis media, sinusitis), head injury.
- **Uncommon acute:** meningitis, encephalitis, raised intracranial pressure, intracranial haemorrhage, hypertension, vasculitis, hunger, dehydration, noise.
- **Common recurrent:** migraine, recurrent headache of childhood, anxiety, depression, attention seeking.
- **Uncommon recurrent** (less than 5% of children with recurrent headache): refractive errors, glaucoma, epilepsy, leukaemia, trigeminal neuralgia, metabolic (lead poisoning, hypoglycaemia, alcohol abuse, glue sniffing).

Clinically. Assess general appearance, and look for evidence of infection. For recurrent or severe persistent headaches check blood pressure, fundi, cranial bruits, head circumference, visual acuity and fields, full neurological assessment.

Investigation. The GP should investigate recurrent or severe persistent headaches with skull X-ray, sinus X-ray, FBC, ESR, serum urea and glucose, urine microscopy and culture. A paediatrician may order lumbar puncture, computerized tomography (CT) scan, cerebral angiography and EEG.

MIGRAINE

Incidence. 1.5% of children by age 7, 4.5% of children by age 15. Boys more than girls before puberty, ratio reversed after puberty.
Aetiology. Familial tendency (80% have an affected parent or sibling). Precipitated by emotion or diet (red wine, chocolate, cheese). Associated with periodic syndrome and travel sickness.

Pathology. Aura and prodromal symptoms are conventionally attributed to intracranial vasoconstriction but may reflect abnormal electrical activity in the cortex. Dilatation of extra-cranial blood vessels causes the headache.

Clinically.

- **Classical migraine**: aura (e.g. fortification spectra), followed by unilateral headache that is severe and throbbing, photophobia, nausea and often vomiting. Headache lasts a few hours.
- **Complicated migraine**: ophthalmoplegia, hemiplegia, ataxia and convulsions starting during the aura of classical migraine.
- **Common migraine**: diffuse headache (relieved by pressure over the temporal arteries), nausea and vomiting. Lasts hours or days.
- **Cluster headache**: sudden pain around one eye associated with ipsilateral sympathetic over-activity (conjunctival injection, tears and a dilated pupil). Headache lasts one hour and repeats many times each day for a few days.

Investigate complicated migraine and migraine associated with symptoms between headaches (anorexia, weight loss, ataxia).

Management. Explain and reassure if appropriate.

- **Treat acute attacks** with buccal (or rectal) prochlorperazine and oral (or rectal) paracetamol. If you give parenteral therapy you will be asked to visit every time the child has a headache. Ergotamine only for common migraine because it can cause complications in classical migraine. Rest in a dark room.
- **Prevention**. Avoid precipitants. If more than 4 attacks per month try prophylactic propranolol or pizotifen. Methysergide if all else fails (only after puberty, only for three months).

Prognosis. Half remit within 5 years.

FAINTS, FITS, AND FUNNY TURNS

- Syncope.
- Hyperventilation.
- Cyanotic breath-holding attacks.
- Acyanotic breath-holding attacks.
- Convulsions.
- Masturbation.
- Night terrors.
- Hypoglycaemia.

SYNCOPE
Definition. Loss of consciousness due to a transient impairment of cerebral blood flow.
Incidence. Vasovagal faints commonly affect adolescent girls.
Aetiology.
1. Commonly vasovagal: peripheral vasodilatation and bradycardia result in hypotension (stress, hunger, pain)
2. Sometimes:
   • Reflex anoxic seizures (vagal asystole in response to pain or fright = acyanotic breatholding attack).
   • Carotid sinus syncope (reflex bradycardia on carotid sinus pressure).
   • Postural hypotension (prolonged standing, side effect of drugs, autonomic neuropathy).
   • Reduced venous return (hypovolaemia, raised intrathoracic pressure with valsalva or whooping cough).
   • Cardiac outflow obstruction causes syncope on exertion (Fallots).
   • Cardiac arrhythmias.
Clinically. Sitting or standing. Suddenly becomes nauseated, giddy and confused. Dim vision and spots in front of the eyes. Pale, cold, sweaty, slow pulse. Collapses for a few seconds or minutes. May convulse if held erect. Recovers without confusion or drowsiness. Between attacks check pulse rate, postural blood pressure, carotid sinus sensitivity, cardiac murmur.
Differential diagnosis of syncope.
1. Hyperventilation and hysteria (tachycardia during collapse).
2. Epilepsy (residual confusion or drowsiness)
3. Hypoglycaemia (gradual onset).
Investigations. Only if history atypical: ECG (with carotid massage), 24 hour ECG, echocardiogram, fasting glucose, EEG with provocation, cardiac electrophysiology.
Treatment. Lie flat on feeling faint.

HYPERVENTILATION
Pathophysiology. Alveolar ventilation in excess of metabolic requirements leads to low carbon dioxide tension in the blood (respiratory alkalosis). This increases protein binding of plasma calcium and a reduced ionised calcium (effective hypocalcaemia).
Incidence. Common in schoolchildren. Girls = boys.
Aetiology. Emotion or habit.
Symptoms. Giddiness, syncope, chest pain, tingling, inability to take a deep and satisfying breath.

Signs. Sighs, irregular thoracic breathing. Chest wall tenderness. Collapse is quite common but tetany is rare. Forced overbreathing often reproduces symptoms.

Investigation. Partial pressure of carbon dioxide < 30 mmHg.

Management. Explain, reassure, reduce any unreasonable stresses. Rebreathing into a paper bag during exacerbations, breathing exercises, hypnotherapy, psychotherapy.

CYANOTIC BREATH HOLDING ATTACKS

Incidence. Common. Age 1 month to 3 years. Children with a low threshold for frustration.

Pathology. Anger – valsalva – raised intrathoracic pressure – reduced venous return to the heart – cyanosis and cerebral anoxia with extended tonic posture and upturned eyes for up to 15 seconds – collapses limp and unconscious – convulsions in predisposed children – starts breathing – complete recovery after 15 seconds.

Management. Distraction at onset of episode. Lie flat in recovery position when collapsed. Do not fuss after recovery. Usually resolves by school age. Increased incidence of syncope in later life.

ACYANOTIC BREATH HOLDING ATTACKS

Incidence. Infants and toddlers. Uncommon.

Clinically. Stimulus (pain) – vagal asystole (pale, limp, unconscious) – may convulse – recover after one minute.

Management. Recovery position to protect airway.

CONVULSIONS

Incidence. 7% of children have one or more convulsions. 1/3 have febrile convulsions and 1/10 have epilepsy.

Aetiology.

- **Age 0-28 days** (neonatal fits): Trauma, hypoglycaemia, hypocalcaemia, CNS malformation.
- **Age 1-6 months**: Infantile spasms, intracranial infection.
- **Age 6 months to 3 years**: febrile convulsions, intracranial infections, breath holding attacks, epilepsy.
- **Age more than 3 years**: epilepsy.

FEBRILE CONVULSIONS

Incidence. 3% of children. Male = female. Age 6 months to 6 years, but usually during second year. Not associated with social class. Associated with: pre-existing neurological abnormality, cerebral problems at birth (20% risk of febrile convulsions), breech delivery, family history of epilepsy or febrile convulsions (15%).

Clinically. Ask for details of the febrile illness, the convulsion, previous development, and previous convulsions. Assess the general condition (sleepy), rectal temperature, meningism (can be present without meningitis).

- **Simple** (80%): generalised grand mal, less than 15 minutes, only one per febrile illness, no focal neurological signs or optic fundus abnormality.
- **Complex** (20%): focal, longer than 15 minutes, more than one per febrile illness, residual neurological deficit.

Management of the acute convulsion. Clear airway, stop the convulsion (rectal diazepam), reduce fever. Admit to hospital except after a simple convulsion in an older child with a family history of febrile convulsions, an obvious infection and unconcerned parents.

Investigations in hospital.
- All children should have FBC, urine analysis (glucose, protein, blood), urine microscopy and culture.
- Sicker children need lumbar puncture (cerebrospinal fluid (CSF) for microscopy and culture), blood biochemistry (calcium, urea, sodium, bilirubin), blood culture.
- After complex or recurrent febrile convulsions check serum for magnesium and lead levels, urine for porphyrins, CT brain scan, ECG, EEG (does not affect prognosis but may suggest another form of seizure).

Management of recurrent convulsions.
- **Discuss** fever control, the use of rectal valium (0.3 mg/kg) and the recovery position. Reassure if appropriate.
- **Prophylaxis** with valproate after the second febrile convulsion for children at increased risk of recurrent febrile convulsions or epilepsy (does not reduce the risk of epilepsy developing). Stop prophylaxis after 2 fit-free years or at age 6.

Prognosis. Simple febrile convulsions do not affect neurological or intellectual development.
- After 1 febrile convulsion, 30% will have another and 10% will have 2 or more.
- Recurrent febrile convulsions are more common if the first febrile convulsion occurred before 18 months or if there is a family history of febrile convulsion.

- After a febrile convulsion 2% of children develop epilepsy. 10% of children with previous neurological abnormalities develop epilepsy.
- Epilepsy is twice as likely after complex febrile convulsions.

EPILEPSY
Definition. A tendency to recurrent seizures.
Incidence. A GP will see a first non-febrile convulsion once a year. 0.5% of children have had a non-febrile convulsion by age 7, and of these 85% have epilepsy. Mentally retarded children frequently have epilepsy. Male = female.
Predisposition:
- 95% idiopathic (familial).
- 5% secondary:
    Perinatal (trauma, hypoxia, jaundice).
    Cerebral infections (meningitis, encephalitis).
    Malformations (vascular, neurofibroma, tuberous sclerosis, hydrocephalus).
    Cerebral tumours.
    Head injury.
    Intracranial haemorrhage.
    Degenerations and metabolic abnormalities.
Precipitants. Fever, exhaustion, trauma, flashing lights, hyperventilation, hypoglycaemia, drugs and drug withdrawal.
Prognosis. Of those with epilepsy 60% have a burst of attacks then remission, 10% have intermittent seizures, 25% have frequent attacks and 5% will be severely disabled.

1. Partial seizures
1(a) Simple focal motor or sensory symptoms without loss of consciousness.
Benign partial epilepsy of childhood. 15% of childhood seizures. Onset age 3-10 years. Male>female. Familial. Simple tonic-clonic spasms of face and hand lasting 60 seconds. Less than one a day. Usually wake the child from sleep. No aura or post-ictal confusion. Easily controlled on carbamazepine or phenytoin. Remits in adolescence. EEG shows unilateral spike waves over the Rolandic area. No anatomical abnormality.
Benign psychomotor epilepsy. Sudden fear and scream followed by salivation, swallowing, pallor and sweating. Lasts 2 minutes responds well to carbamazepine and remits in adolescence.

1(b) Complex focal motor or sensory symptoms followed by loss of consciousness = **Psychomotor epilepsy** (Temporal lobe epilepsy).

Common. Stare – automatisms (organised movements such as lip smacking), hallucinations (smell, taste, vision, deja vu), mood changes – collapse. Lasts 10 seconds. Temporal lobe spikes on EEG. Aetiology: temporal lobe sclerosis, cyst or tumour. Treat with carbamazepine and/or phenytoin and/or neurosurgery. Prognosis: 33% remit, 33% become independent on medication, 33% need institutional care and 5% die in childhood. Psychiatric disorders are common.

1(c). Partial seizures with secondary generalisation. 70% of childhood epilepsy. Usually starts before age 5. Often have cerebral palsy or mental retardation. Aura (sensory, psychic or autonomic) – generalised tonic clonic convulsion with loss of consciousness. EEG shows inter-ictal focal paroxysms. Resistant to anticonvulsants. Prognosis is worse if the epilepsy is severe or there is mental handicap, neurological abnormality or a structural lesion.

2. Generalised seizures

2(a). Petit mal. 10% of childhood epilepsy. Age 3 to 13. Female > male. Familial. No structural abnormality. 'Absence' for less than 10 seconds at a time more than 10 times each day. Patient unaware. Normal IQ but frequent seizures cause learning difficulties. EEG show 3 Hz spike and wave pattern precipitated by hyperventilation. Easily controlled on valproate or ethosuximide. Remits in adult life but 30% develop grand mal.

Differential Diagnosis of blank appearance without collapse.
• Day-dreaming, masturbation.
• Incomplete syncope.
• Epilepsy:
    • Typical petit mal.
    • Atypical petit mal (onset in adolescence, atypical EEG).
    • Temporal lobe epilepsy (episodes last longer than petit mal and occur less often. There is an aura, complex automatisms, and post-ictal confusion).
    • Simple partial seizures (last 60 seconds, less than 1 per day).

2(b) Grand mal (Primary generalized convulsive epilepsy).
Incidence. Uncommon. Onset after age 5. Associated with petit mal. Not associated with neurological or organic psychiatric abnormalities.

Clinically. No aura. Tonic spasm with collapse, loss of consciousness, cyanosis – after 60 seconds clonic spasms with incontinence and tongue biting – after 3 minutes coma – gradual recovery after minutes or hours with headache, drowsiness, confusion, myalgia and automatisms. Status epilepticus is a series of major seizures without intervening recovery of consciousness.

Investigations. EEG may show bursts of spike waves between seizures; diffuse runs of spike waves in tonic phase; slow waves alternating with spike waves in the clonic phase.

Prognosis. Seizure free remission in 70% of patients on monotherapy (carbamazepine, phenytoin, phenobarbitone). After 15 years 80% remain in remission off treatment.

2(c) **Myoclonic** (brief jerks of an extremity or brief atonia).

Infantile spasms (West's syndrome, hypsarrhythmia, salaam attacks). Uncommon. Onset age 4–9 months. 70% have localised or diffuse brain lesions (10% tuberous sclerosis, 10% have brain malformations, 10% chronic trauma), 30% are cryptogenic. No association with pertussis vaccination.

Symptoms. Sudden flexion of trunk, head and arms. Lasts 1 second but can occur several times a minute.

Management. CT scan. EEG shows hypsarrhythmia. Try prednisolone or ACTH for three months then benzodiazepines or valproate.

Prognosis. Children with brain damage are refractory to treatment and develop severe psychomotor retardation by age 5. Cryptogenic cases respond better to therapy, seizures settle at age 5 and half develop a normal IQ.

Myoclonic astatic epilepsy. Uncommon, onset age 2–7 years. Frequent falls due to brief myoclonus or atonia (Drop attacks). Develop psychomotor retardation. Refractory to treatment (benzodiazepines, corticosteroids and ketogenic diet). In adult life 5% have a full remission, 20% have infrequent fits on medication, the others are severely disabled.

Benign myoclonic epilepsy of infancy. Seizures mimic infantile spasms but occur less frequently. Controlled by valproate. Inter-ictal EEG is normal. All remit in childhood.

Juvenile myoclonic epilepsy. Onset after age 5. Bilateral single or repetitive jerks typically affecting arms on waking or going to sleep. Photosensitive. Associated with grand mal. Bursts of polyspike waves on EEG. Only 10% remit but the remainder are fit-free on valproate.

INVOLUNTARY MOVEMENTS

The basal ganglia coordinate automatic and voluntary movement. A predominance of dopaminergic pathways results in hyperkinetic dyskinesias (tics, chorea, hemiballismus, tardive dyskinesias) which are absent when asleep, worse when anxious and associated with restlessness and reduced tone but normal tendon reflexes. Weak dopaminergic pathways result in hypokinetic dyskinesias (Parkinsonism, dystonia) which are relieved by L-dopa and associated with increased tone.

TICS
Definition. Stereotypic, repetitive, involuntary movements.
Aetiology.
1. **Simple developmental tics** affect 15% of primary school children. Familial. Movements affect head, neck and shoulders (blinking, sniffing). Helped by avoiding stresses such as parental demands to stop 'doing it'. May require relaxation exercises, psychotherapy, behaviour therapy. Stop in adolescence.
2. **Manneristic tics** in mentally retarded or autistic children. Rocking, head banging, self mutilation.
3. **Multiple tics** due to dopamine releasing drugs, SSPE, Gilles de la Tourette syndrome. Helped by haloperidol.

CHOREA
Definition. Non-repetitive involuntary movements that are purposeless, jerky and interrupt voluntary and automatic movements. Principally affect axial and proximal limb muscles. Tongue cannot be held protruded. Hemiballismus is a severe form of unilateral chorea.
Aetiology. Usually dyskinetic cerebral palsy. Sometimes: drug induced chorea, Sydenham's chorea, chorea minima (mild chorea in a normal child), familial (Wilson's disease).
Management. see dyskinetic cerebral palsy.

ATHETOSIS
Definition. Slow, writhing involuntary movements that are worse during voluntary movements.
Aetiology. Usually cerebral palsy or drug induced (phenothiazines). Sometimes idiopathic or associated with congenital malformations, brain degenerations (Wilson's disease).
Management. See cerebral palsy.

DYSTONIA
Frozen athetotic postures.

TARDIVE DYSKINESIA
Facial contortions caused by prolonged treatment with phenothiazines, haloperidol, carbamazepine, L-dopa. Typically chewing and grimaces. Do not stop on withdrawing the medication.

TREMOR
Definition. Fine rhythmic movements of the head and limbs.
Aetiology.
* Physiological + tired, anxious, on medication (salbutamol, lithium, phenytoin, valproate, theophylline and caffeine).
* Benign essential tremor. Dominant inheritance. Starts in early childhood and gets worse but rarely incapacitates. Helped by alcohol, propranolol and diazepam.
* Withdrawal of phenobarbitone etc
* Metabolic: hepatic failure, uraemia, thyrotoxic, hypoglycaemic.
* Intracranial lesions: Parkinson's syndrome, encephalitis, cerebellar tumours.

Parkinson's syndrome
= tremor, difficulty initiating movements (bradykinesia) and flexor rigidity. Rare in children. Aetiology: drug induced >> post-encephalitic, SSPE. Prescribe L-dopa with a peripheral decarboxylase inhibitor to reduce peripheral side effects.

HYPOTONIA

Floppy babies lie like frogs when supine. In ventral suspension the limbs and head hang limply. The limbs are hypermobile when shaken. Reflexes are depressed or absent. Spontaneous movements are reduced. Muscles feel soft and may fasciculate. The infant and young child show delayed gross motor development.
Aetiology.
* **Acute neonatal hypotonia**: prematurity, drugs taken by the mother (alcohol, benzodiazepines, pethidine), perinatal hypoxia or trauma, metabolic problems (hypoglycaemia, hypocalcaemia, hypokalaemia, hyponatraemia, hypomagnesaemia, acidosis), infection.

- **Acute infantile hypotonia**: any infection, metabolic disorders, drugs, polyneuritis (Guillain-Barré), spinal muscular atrophy, poliomyelitis.
- **Chronic hypotonia in the infant and young child**: mental retardation, cerebral palsy, hyperextensibility syndrome, muscular dystrophy, congenital myopathies, spinal muscular atrophy myaesthenia, metabolic disorders (storage diseases, porphyria, rickets).

Investigation. Refer for infection screen (culture blood, urine, CSF), CxR, FBC, metabolic screen. CSF for protein. Cerebral ultrasound for neonate. If still no diagnosis: creatinine phosphokinase, EMG, muscle biopsy, sural nerve biopsy, nerve conduction studies, EEG.

MUSCULAR DYSTROPHY
Definition. After a period of apparently normal development, there is a progressive degeneration of muscles due to an inherited abnormality of the muscles themselves.

Duchene muscular dystrophy
Epidemiology. Affects 20/100,000 live male births each year. At any one time there are only 1,500 affected children in the UK. Sex linked recessive but 1/3 are spontaneous mutations.
Clinically. Onset age 1 to 4. Weakness and contractures of the trunk and proximal limb muscles, intercostal muscles and myocardium. Average IQ is 85. Die in teens with chest infections, heart failure or heart block.
Investigations. CPK is very high (>1,000 iu/l) in affected children and raised in 70% of carriers.
Management. Genetic counselling. Exercise and weight limiting diet. Percutaneous tenotomies and passive physiotherapy to reduce disability from contractures.

Limb girdle dystrophy
Autosomal recessive affecting 7/100,000 live births. Onset age 10-30. Weak shoulder and pelvic girdle without contractures. In wheelchair after 20 years, but lifespan normal. IQ normal. CPK normal.

Facio-scapulo-humeral dystrophy
Autosomal dominant affecting 4/million live births. Onset age 10-40. Expressionless face, weak shoulder girdle and upper arm. IQ normal. Normal lifespan. CPK is usually normal.

Myotonia congenita

Autosomal dominant. Rare. Presents as neonate with odd cry who has difficulty feeding and opening his eyes. Tonic contraction produces massive muscles that are stiff when cold. Improves with age. Helped by quinidine and procainamide. Normal IQ and lifespan.

Congenital myopathies (Benign congenital hypotonia)

Rare. Inherited (often autosomal dominant). Classified by histological or ultrastructural defect. Severe cases present with a floppy baby but most start as a non-progressive limb girdle weakness that initially delays gross motor development then improves in later childhood. There is no fasciculation. Diagnosis made on muscle biopsy. CPK and EMG are normal.

SPINAL MUSCULAR ATROPHY (SMA)

Rare. Autosomal recessive. Death of anterior horn cells results in atrophy of groups of myocytes. CSF, nerve conduction studies and CPK are normal. Muscle biopsy confirms diagnosis suggested by EMG. Antenatal diagnosis is not available. Physiotherapy, tenotomies and appliances can reduce handicap.
Classification.
1. **Acute infantile SMA (Werdnig Hoffman disease)**: floppy baby dies in infancy with severe contractures, respiratory infections and hypoventilation.
2. **Chronic infantile SMA**: weakness develops in late infancy. Live for years with moderately severe weakness and contractures.
3. **Juvenile SMA (Kugelberg Welander syndrome)**: limb girdle weakness from early childhood. Often live into sixth decade.

GUILLAIN-BARRÉ SYNDROME

Rapid onset of symmetrical weakness and hypotonia over days or weeks. Often show meningism. Polyneuritis, but sensory system spared. CSF protein is high with a normal cell count.

MYAESTHENIA

Definition. Abnormal fatiguability of muscle due to impaired neuromuscular conduction.
Classification.
1. **Juvenile myaesthenia gravis** affects 1 in a million adolescents (4/5 female). Resembles the adult disease with thymitis and IgG anti-receptor antibody. Muscle fatigue is reversed by anticholinesterase.

2. **Infantile myaesthenia.** Very rare. Often familial (autosomal recessive). No anti-receptor antibodies. Non-progressive weakness of extra-ocular muscles.
3. **Passive myaesthenia gravis.** Very rare. 1/6 of infants born to women with myaesthenia gravis are affected by maternal antibodies which have crossed the placenta.
4. **Drug induced myaesthenia** (gentamycin).
5. **Symptomatic myaesthenia** (leukaemia).

HYPERTONIA

Hypertonic babies are jittery with an odd cry, feeding difficulties, and increased resistance to passive movement (clasp knife rigidity with pyramidal lesion; lead pipe or cogwheel rigidity with extrapyramidal lesion). Brisk tendon reflexes, upgoing plantar reflexes (can be normal up to age 2). Delayed motor development. Lie with legs extended and scissored, but arms adducted and elbows hyperflexed. May develop contractures or involuntary movements.
Aetiology.
- Pyramidal lesion: cerebral palsy, brainstem tumour, hydrocephalus, multiple sclerosis, spinal cord compression.
- Extrapyramidal: Parkinson's syndrome, Jacob-creutzfeldt disease.
- Other: tetany, tetanus.

CEREBRAL PALSY
Definition. A disorder of posture and movement resulting from a non-progressive lesion of the developing brain before or during the neonatal period. The expression of the lesion changes as the brain matures.
Incidence. 1/500 live births.
- 70% spastic (lesion in cortex or internal capsule).
- 20% dyskinetic (lesion in basal ganglia).
- 10% ataxic (lesion in cerebellum).
Aetiology.
The relative importance of the various causes of cerebral palsy is hotly debated in medical literature and courts of law.
- 35% cryptogenic.
- 30% perinatal insult (many of these may be cryptogenic).
- 20% genetic.
- 10% postnatal disease (meningitis, encephalitis, trauma, stroke).
- 5% intra-uterine infection, irradiation or drug induced damage.

Management.
- **Prevention.** Good obstetric care.
- **Early diagnosis.** Developmental surveillance
- **Physiotherapy.** Position to reduce hypertonia and prevent contractures. Encourage symmetrical movement/awareness of limbs. Brace to allow walking.
- **Aids and appliances.** Splints and braces. Wheelchairs. Possum.
- **Surgery.** Tenotomies for contractures. Femoral derotation osteotomy to enable a diplegic to walk. Neurotomy to relieve spasm.
- **Education.** Academic, speech training, social skills, vocational.
- **Support the carers.**
- **Drugs.** Antispasmodics.

Spastic hemiplegia
Risk factors. Maternal eclamptic toxaemia (50%), premature (40%), postmature (20%), fetal distress in labour (25%), birth trauma, neonatal apnoea/cyanosis/fits/hypothermia (80%), hydrocephalus.

Pathology. Infarct of cortex or internal capsule. Weakness affects the arm more than the leg (in the primary motor cortex the leg area is supplied by the anterior and middle cerebral arteries whereas the arm area, which is more lateral, is only supplied by the middle cerebral). The trunk and face which have bilateral cortical representation are relatively spared. The weakness is more evident distally. Voluntary movements are weak but involuntary reflex movements are strong.

Clinically. Neonate feeds poorly but sleeps well Asymmetrical tone and reduced spontaneous movements in the affected limbs. Motor milestones are delayed. The limbs on one side are smaller, colder and spastic.

Prognosis. Almost all walk by school age. 30% have an IQ less than 70, 40% have hemisensory loss, 10% have hemianopia and 50% have epilepsy.

Differential diagnosis of hemiplegia.
- Cerebral palsy (abnormal development since the neonatal period)
- Intracranial infection (encephalitis, meningitis, abscess, AIDS)
- Intracranial vascular accident (accidental or nonaccidental injury, migraine, epilepsy, embolus).
- Intracranial mass (tumour, aneurysm).
- Hydrocephalus.
- Rarely: cerebral degenerations, multiple sclerosis.
- Disorder of the limb (fracture).

Spastic diplegia and quadriplegia

Risk factors. Mother with a poor obstetric history, maternal alcoholism, intrauterine infection (rubella, CMV, toxoplasmosis), prematurity, familial spastic diplegia.

Pathology. Periventricular infarction.

Clinically. Neonate is dystonic. Infant develops flexor hypertonus.

Prognosis.

* In diplegia the legs are far more severely affected than the arms, 10% have mental handicap, and 10% have fits.
* In quadriplegia the arms are as spastic as the legs, all are mentally retarded, 50% have fits, 30% are blind (optic atrophy or cortical blindness), 50% have squints. Pseudobulbar palsy is common (eating and speech severely affected, chronic otitis media).

Differential diagnosis of quadriplegia and diplegia.

* Cerebral palsy
* Damage to spinal cord or cauda equina (syringomyelia)

Dyskinetic cerebral palsy

Pathology. The neurones of the basal ganglia are selectively damaged by neonatal jaundice (bilirubin poisons mitochondria) and hypoxaemia (placental insufficiency, ante-partum haemorrhage, prolapsed cord).

Clinically.

* After hypoxia: the neonate is hypotonic, needs help with breathing, and feeds poorly. He commonly has convulsions and may die. Infants who survive the neonatal period remain irritable, unresponsive and difficult to feed. Spasticity, choreoathetosis, dystonia, bulbar palsy, mental retardation and microcephaly develop after the fifth month.
* After jaundice: the neonate has extensor spasms, sunsetting eyes, and doggy-paddling movements. He may die with apnoea or hyperpyrexia. Dystonia dvelops after the fifth month. Athetosis develops after infancy.

Prognosis. 50% have a low IQ, epilepsy is uncommon. Eventually learns to walk. Often deaf.

Ataxic cerebral palsy

Due to lesions of the cerebellum, its inputs (vestibular, proprioceptive, visual) or output tracts (to basal ganglia and cortex).

Familial dysfunction without anatomical abnormality.

Congenital malformation (cerebellar hypoplasia, hydrocephalus).

Perinatal cerebral insult (jaundice, hypothyroidism, hypoxia, intracranial haemorrhage or ischaemia).

Clinically. Hypotonia, mild weakness, pendulous tendon reflexes. Truncal and volitional ataxia

ATAXIA AND CLUMSY CHILDREN

Clumsiness. A clumsy child is one whose motor development lags behind their general abilities by two years or more.

Ataxia. Severe clumsiness = inco-ordination of posture and gait (truncal ataxia) or hand movements and speech (volitional ataxia).

Truncal ataxia. The infant is floppy and slightly weak but tendon reflexes are present and often pendulous. Delayed motor milestones. Eventually walks with a broad based gait.

Volitional ataxia. Hand movements are jerky, intention tremor demonstrated by the finger-nose pointing test. Mild hypotonia. Difficulty in learning complex motor skills shows as immature speech and dyspraxia. Nystagmus and slurred speech are more typical of acquired ataxias than congenital ataxias.

Vertigo. A feeling that you or the surroundings are rotating. A consequence of damage to the inner ear, vestibular nerve or its central connections. Usually associated with truncal ataxia and nausea. Young children have difficulty expressing this symptom.

Pathology. Ataxia results from abnormalities of:
- The cerebellum.
- Its inputs (vestibular nerve, eyes, proprioceptive fibres in the spino-cerebellar tracts, cerebral cortex).
- Its outputs (cerebral cortex, extra-pyramidal motor system).

Aetiology.

Chronic non-progressive ataxia
- Normal variation or delayed motor maturation (? familial).
- Minimal brain dysfunction.
- Mental retardation.
- Cerebral palsy.

Chronic progressive ataxia
- Repetitive head injury.
- Raised intracranial pressure (intracranial tumours, hydrocephalus).
- Metabolic: hypothyroidism.
- Rarely: hereditary degenerations (Friedreich's ataxia), spinal cord disease, peripheral neuropathy.

Acute ataxia

- Para-infectious (chickenpox).
- Meningitis, encephalitis.
- Vestibular problems: viral vestibulitis, otitis media.
- Toxic and metabolic (hypoglycaemia, phenytoin toxicity, lead toxicity, alcohol abuse, glue sniffing, aminoacidurias).
- Head injury may cause ataxia lasting months.
- Cerebrovascular accidents.
- Multiple sclerosis.

Differential diagnosis of ataxia.

- Involuntary movements.
- Weakness.
- Visual problems: severe myopia, visuo-spatial difficulties.
- Emotional distress.

Friedreich's ataxia

Epidemiology. Uncommon. The commonest cause of primary neuronal degeneration. Autosomal recessive. 5% of the normal population are carriers.

Clinically. Starts aged 8-12 with truncal and volitional ataxia (loss of spino-cerebellar tracts). Then:

Weakness and wasting start distally (loss of cortico-spinal tracts). Characteristically tendon reflexes are absent despite extensor plantars. Pes cavus (55%). Scoliosis (80%).

Loss of position and vibration sense (loss of posterior columns).

Dysarthria (100%), optic nerve atrophy (30%), deafness (10%).

Cardiomyopathy (40% are symptomatic).

Prognosis. Diabetes (10%). Chairbound in twenties. Dead by middle age.

Minimal brain dysfunction syndrome

Epidemiology. Common. May be a mild form of cerebral palsy. Often familial. No metabolic or anatomical abnormality.

Clinically. Minor abnormalities on neurological or psychological testing.

Clumsy = mild ataxia (falls), involuntary movements, sensory inattention, impaired spatial awareness.

Learning difficulties: dyslexia, dysgraphia, easily distracted, difficulty understanding abstract concepts, poor memory.

Behavioural problems arise because they are unable to meet the expectations of their parents, siblings, friends and teachers. Stuttering, shyness, enuresis, conduct disorders, hyperactivity.

Management. See chapter on 'Education' for guidelines on the care of children with 'Special Educational Needs'. See chapter on 'Psychiatry' for guidelines on the care of behavioural problems.

Differential diagnosis of 'slow and unsteady'.
• Simple developmental delay.
• Minimal brain dysfunction.
• Any of the causes of ataxia.
• Emotional stress.
• Social deprivation.
• Simple mental retardation.
• Specific learning difficulties.
• Epilepsy.

MENTAL RETARDATION

Definition. Mental retardation is a global delay in the development of cognitive learning (contrast learning by repetition without understanding). Intelligence tests attempt to compare a subject's general ability to the average for a child of his age. This ratio is the Intelligence Quotient (IQ).
• **Severe subnormality** is a state of arrested or incomplete development of mind which includes subnormality of intelligence and is of such a degree and nature that the patient is incapable of living an independent life or of guarding himself against serious exploitation (Mental Health Act of 1959). About 0.3% of children have an IQ<50 = severely subnormal. Of these 30% have Down's syndrome and 30% need institutional care.
• **Subnormality** is a state of mind that can be improved by training (Mental Health Act of 1959). About 3% of children have an IQ<70 (2 standard deviations below the mean) = Subnormal.
Incidence. A GP will diagnose one new case of subnormality nearly every year and one new case of severe subnormality every 10 years. He will have 60 subnormal people on his list.
Aetiology.
• **Severe subnormality** is not associated with social class:
  • Brain damage: cerebral palsy, infection, haematoma, child abuse.
  • Congenital abnormality (hydrocephalus).
  • Epilepsy (infantile spasms).
  • Syndromes: chromosomal disorders (Down's), metabolic abnormalities endocrine abnormalities (hypothyroid), Duchenne muscular dystrophy.

- **Subnormality** is usually due to sub-cultural mental retardation. Strongly associated with socio-economic class IV and V. The psychopathic or mentally retarded parents regard the child as normal. Mild or moderate mental retardation. Normal motor development and appearance.

Differential diagnosis of mental retardation.

- Relative mental retardation: a child with IQ>70 may be treated as mentally handicapped by more intelligent parents and siblings.
- Specific learning disorders (dyslexia, dyspraxia).
- Psychosocial deprivation.
- Sensory defect (blind, deaf).
- Psychiatric problem (depression > autism).
- Epilepsy.
- Toxic effects of medications or drugs of abuse.
- Dementia.

Prevention.

- Rubella immunisation before conception.
- Avoid drugs starting prior to conception (cigarettes, alcohol).
- Antenatal diagnosis and selective abortion.
- Atraumatic delivery.
- Supervision of children in disorganized families by health visitors and social workers.

Screening.

- Neonatal blood test for PKU (Guthrie test) and TSH.
- Child health surveillance (funny looking kid, delayed motor development (85%), retarded speech development).

Referral of children with suspected subnormality.

- Subnormality: refer for assessment of educational needs.
- Severe subnormality: refer to a paediatric neurologist for exclusion of a treatable cause.

Education.

- Formal remedial education is more stressful than normal social interaction with parents and siblings who are aware of the special needs of the mentally retarded child. It is better to read to him than make him fail at reading.
- Encourage development in areas least affected by handicap (usually motor skills).
- Train in acceptable behaviour patterns. Although cognitive learning is impaired pavlovian conditioning can be used to teach the activities of everyday living.

Medical care. 80% of severely subnormal people have major medical problems.

Social support.

- Support for the family: financial support, listening, consistent information from involved professionals, holiday and crisis admissions for the child.
- Institutional care is provided for 50,000 people. The Mental Health Act 1983 encouraged small units with varying degrees of independence. This initiative has been limited by funding. The district handicap team co-ordinates the care of children. In some areas there are equivalent teams for adults.

DOWN'S SYNDROME (TRISOMY 21)

Incidence. 1/700 live births. Risk increases with maternal age 1/1500 at age 25, 1/350 at age 35, 1/100 at age 40. After one child affected by simple Trisomy 21 the risk of recurrence is 1%.

Aetiology: 92% - simple Trisomy 21; 5% - translocations (often familial; 3% mosaics.

The syndrome. Floppy baby. Short child with characteristic face (small head, flat nose, sloping eyes), short neck, umbilical hernia (hypotonia), short limbs, spade-like hands and feet, poorly developed genitalia and delayed appearance of secondary sexual characteristics. Severe mental subnormality.

Associated with:

- Infections of skin and otitis media.
- Visual problems: squint (33%), myopia (33%), nystagmus (15%), keratoconus (6%), cataract (1%). 5% become blind.
- Deafness: glue ear is very common, sensorineural deafness is 3 times commoner than normal.
- Cardiac abnormalities (30%): ASD, VSD, PDA.
- Gut abnormalities (5%): duodenal atresia, anal atresia, pyloric stenosis.
- Leukaemia (1%).
- Hypothyroidism in 1% of infants and 17% of adults. All autoimmune diseases are commoner.
- Orthopaedic problems: congenital dislocation of hip.
- Males are sub-fertile and 14% have undescended testes.

Prognosis. 75% survive to 5 years and 50% to middle age. Mean IQ<40. Social skills are often good for a given IQ but 13% develop serious behaviour problems.

SPEECH DELAY and SPECIFIC LEARNING DEFECTS
See chapter on 'Education'.

SMALL HEAD

Differential diagnosis.
- Small head of a normal child. By definition, 3% of normal children will have a head circumference below the 3rd centile.
- Small head of an abnormally small child.
- Small brain (microcephaly) of severe mental retardation.
- Anencephaly.
- Craniosynostosis. Premature fusion of the skull sutures results in a small, deformed skull. Brain growth is arrested. Raised intracranial pressure causes fits, mental retardation and optic atrophy.

Clinically. Be suspicious of an odd looking child, delayed development, poor feeding, head circumference crossing centiles or disproportionate to body.

Management. Reassure a small child of small parents who has normal features and a head circumference growing along a constant centile line (normal growth velocity). If the parents are still worried or the child does not meet these criteria, arrange a skull X-ray, cerebral ultrasound or CT scan.

BIG HEAD

Differential diagnosis.
- Big head of a big normal child. By definition, 3% of normal children will have a head circumference above the 97th centile.
- Big head of an abnormally big child = gigantism.
- Hydrocephalus.
- Hydrancephaly = anencephaly with a cerebral cyst.
- Big brain (megalencephaly): cryptogenic, storage diseases.
- Subdural haematoma or abscess.
- Intracranial tumour.

HYDROCEPHALUS

Definition. Dilatation of the ventricles due to excessive CSF pressure.

Incidence. Present in 1/1000 neonates. Develops in another 1/1000 children. A GP will see 1 new case every 12 years. Risk factors:
- Family history of hydrocephalus. If one child is affected, subsequent children have 50/1,000 incidence of hydrocephalus.
- Hydramnios.
- Neonates and children who have required intensive care.
- Children with neurological problems especially meningomyelocele.

Aetiology.
- **Overproduction of CSF** is rare.
- **Obstruction to the flow of CSF through the ventricles** (non-communicating hydrocephalus):
  - Malformations cause 45% of infantile hydrocephalus. The commonest malformation is the Arnold Chiari Malformation of the cerebellum which blocks the outflow of the fourth ventricle.
  - Infection, haemorrhage, tumour.
- **Obstruction to CSF flow in the subarachnoid space** or impaired resorption of CSF by the arachnoid granulations (communicating hydrocephalus): subarachnoid haemorrhage, meningitis.

Clinically.
- Chronic hydrocephalus: head circumference on a higher centile than weight and height. Tense fontanelle. On percussion the skull is resonant or like a cracked pot (delayed closure of sutures). Down-turned eyes ('setting-sun'). Papilloedema. Optic atrophy. Mental retardation or dementia. Spasticity. Epilepsy.
- Acute hydrocephalus (rare) causes headache, vomiting, papilloedema and drowsiness.

Investigation.
- Skull X-ray may suggest, and ultrasound may confirm the diagnosis but CT scan defines the pathology.
- Ventricular CSF pressure monitoring is the most accurate way to assess the activity of hydrocephalus.

Treatment.
- Carbonic anhydrase inhibitors and isosorbide dinitrate may reduce CSF pressure for a while.
- Definitive surgery of the causative lesion if possible.
- CSF shunt (ventriculoperitoneal > ventriculovenous).

Complications of CSF shunts.
- **All**: the ventricles may collapse if there is excessive drainage, the shunt acts as a focus for epilepsy or infection, the top end may block off causing acute hydrocephalus, CSF may leak around the shunt.
- **Those draining into the peritoneal space**: peritonitis, perforation of bowel, occlusion by omentum.
- **Those draining into the vena cava**: thrombosis occluding the shunt or vein, pulmonary embolism, bacteraemia and SBE.

Prognosis. 30% die in childhood. 30% are moderately or severely mentally retarded. 30% of those with shunts have epilepsy.

SPINA BIFIDA (SB)

Definition. Failure of fusion of the vertebral arches.
Incidence. Spina bifida occulta affects 50% of children, meningocele affects 0.03%, myelomeningocele affects 0.3%. A GP will see one new case of meningocele or myelomeningocele every 6 years. Risk factors include:
- Family history. After 1 child with SB the next child has a 5% risk of SB. Vitamin supplements taken from before conception may reduce the risk of recurrence.
- Season. Autumn babies.
- Race. Caucasian.
- Lower socio-economic class.
- Maternal vitamin deficiency.

Pathology.
Spina bifida occulta: the bony arch is split (L5, S1) but the meninges lie within the vertebral canal. The skin is intact but there may be a naevus or pit. Rare children with associated malformations of the spinal cord or vertebrae develop neurological defects.

Meningocele: the meninges protrude from the vertebral canal. The skin is intact. Rarely symptomatic. 20% also have hydrocephalus due to an Arnold Chiari malformation.

Myelomeningocele: the unfolded spinal cord is exposed in the thoraco-lumbar region. Infection of the spinal cord is the usual cause of death. The neurological deficit depends on the anatomy of the lesion but weakness, anaesthesia and loss of bladder and bowel function are common. There are always other abnormalities: hydrocephalus (90%), anencephaly, hemivertebrae, absent ribs, urinary tract malformations.

Management.
- **Spina bifida occulta**. Sinogram if a dermal sinus is deep.
- **Meningocele**. Surgical skin closure in the neonatal period.
- **Myelomeningocele**. Incubator. Neonates with mild neurological defects and no serious associated abnormalities should have early surgery to close the skin over the lesion (70% survive to adult life). If the lesion is simply covered with a sterile gauze dressing soaked in saline the exposed cord epithelializes after a few months (30% live to adult life). Of those who survive early infancy: 6% are normal, 40% are self caring (moderate IQ and walk with calipers), 39% require multi-disciplinary care for the rest of their lives, 15% are bedridden, severely mentally handicapped and incontinent.

ACUTE CLOUDING OF CONSCIOUSNESS

Differential diagnosis in order of decreasing frequency:
• Head injury.
• Infections: meningitis and encephalitis.
• Cerebral anoxia.
• Epileptic status.
• Intracranial haemorrhage or space occupying lesion.
• Toxic or metabolic encephalopathy.

HEAD INJURY
Aetiology. Accidents > non-accidental injury or birth trauma.
Management. Find out how the injury occurred. Assess and record level of consciousness. Identify other significant injuries.
• Minimal trauma. No bump. Advise parents to bring the child back if worried (vomiting, unusual drowsiness, or limb weakness).
• A bump on the head. Impaired consciousness for less than 20 minutes after trauma. Alert. No focal signs. Normal Skull X-ray. Advise parents to bring the child back if worried.
• Impaired consciousness for more than 20 minutes, sleepy, or focal signs. Transfer to casualty.
• Coma: airway, breathing, circulation. Transfer to casualty.

MENINGITIS
Incidence. 1500 cases per year. Commonest in infancy. 1/1000 children have had meningitis by age 5, after which it is much less common. Viral meningitis is commoner than bacterial meningitis.
Aetiology.
Neonates: E. coli, Streptococcus pyogenes.
Acute viral: mumps, coxsackie, echovirus.
Acute bacterial: meningococcal, H. influenzae, pneumococcal.
Chronic: tuberculous meningitis (30 children per year in Britain).
Clinically. Infants stop feeding and the fontanelle bulges. Children may have fever, headache, neck stiffness, prostration, and vomiting. Convulsions, cranial nerve palsies, confusion, drowsiness or coma are less common than in encephalitis. Purpuric rash suggests meningococcal septicaemia.
Management.
• Admit to hospital. If meningococcal meningitis is suspected give i.v. benzyl penicillin before admission. Otherwise, the antibiotic can be selected on the basis of the CSF microscopy.

- Prophyactic antibiotics are reserved for 'kissing' contacts. In practice this includes parents, siblings, childminders and medical staff who actually handled the child. Antibiotics are given for three days. Throat swabs merely generate panic and guilt because at any instant 10-30% of healthy people carry meningococcus in their throats.
- Immunisation with polyvalent pneumococcal vaccine for those at high risk.

Prognosis.
Viral meningitis is seldom fatal. A few children are left with hearing impairment or learning difficulties.
Bacterial meningitis kills 10% of those affected and leaves 25% with major defects: brain damage, deafness.

ENCEPHALITIS
Incidence. 1,000 cases per year in Britain. Age 5-11 years.
Aetiology.
- Infective: herpes viruses. Presents like meningitis but convulsions, cranial nerve palsies, confusion, drowsiness or coma are common. If herpes simplex is suspected give acyclovir. 50% die and half of the survivors are severely handicapped.
- Post infectious: measles. Towards the end of a viral illness the child develops a progressive encephalitis. 10% die despite supportive treatment. 50% of the survivors are handicapped.
- Chronic encephalitis: SSPE affects up to 5 children each year in Britain. Intellectual deterioration precedes choreoathetosis and epilepsy. Death usually occurs within 1 year.

INTRACRANIAL SPACE OCCUPYING LESIONS
Classification.
- Neoplasms.
- Malformations.
- Abscess.
- Haematoma.

Clinically. Often present like hydrocephalus. Ataxia, tremor, nystagmus, and contralateral hemiparesis are common with cerebellar lesions. Cranial nerve lesions, drowsiness and pupillary abnormalities are a late sign indicating brain stem compression.
Investigation. As described for hydrocephalus.
Treatment. Surgical excision.

Neoplasms

200 children are affected each year in the UK. A GP will diagnose one case if he lives 1,000 years. 70% are below the tentorium. Often present with raised intracranial pressure (headache, ataxia).

- Cerebellar astrocytoma.
- Medulloblastoma.
- Haemangioblastoma.
- Gliomas: pontine, supratentorial.
- Pituitary tumours: adenoma, craniopharyngioma.

Malformations

- Tuberous sclerosis (See chapter on 'Dermatology').
- Neurofibromatosis (See chapter on 'Dermatology').
- Sturge-Weber syndrome (See chapter on 'Dermatology').
- Anencephaly. Affects 1 in every 1,000 births in Britain. Females (3:1). The forebrain, midbrain, skull vault and overlying skin are absent. Associated with hydramnios, premature delivery, and spina bifida. Seldom survive more than a few days. Affects 5% of subsequent children born to the same parents.
- Hydranencephaly. The cerebral cortex is replaced by fluid. Die as neonates.
- Megalencephaly. Rare. The cerebral hemispheres are enlarged.

Brain abscess

Rare. Caused by S. aureus and anaerobes. Usually associated with congenital heart disease or mastoiditis. The signs of an intracranial space occupying lesion are combined with a fever. Surgical drainage and antibiotics. Epilepsy is very common after an abscess has healed.

DEMENTIA

Definition. Gradual deterioration in intellect. Presents as slow development but leads to the loss of acquired skills. Often associated with ataxia, involuntary movements, epilepsy.

Aetiology.

- Metabolic abnormalities (Wilson's disease).
- Chronic brain infections (SSPE).
- Hereditary cerebral degenerations (Huntingdon's chorea). A GP will see 1 new case every 1,500 years of practice.
- Drugs and poisons.
- Progressive anatomical abnormalities (hydrocephalus).

17. EYES

VISION TESTING
You must be practised in using the following tests:
- Neonate: copying facial expressions; following a light; red reflex.
- 6 weeks: cover/uncover test to exclude squint.
- 7 months: rolling balls, rotating drum (opticokinetic nystagmus).
- 3 years: matching letters (Sheridan Gardiner test card).
- 5 years: Snellen chart. Acuity = the distance (metres) the patient was standing from the chart divided by the distance at which a normal person could read the smallest letter distinguished by the patient.

REFRACTIVE DISORDERS
Refraction can be tested in older children by asking them to read through different lenses, slotted into spectacle frames, until the test type is seen clearly. Pre-school children can be tested during fundoscopy by interposing lenses between the dilated eye of the child and the ophthalmoscope.

Hypermetropia. Significant only when extreme (uncommon). The eyeball is too short, making it difficult to focus on near objects.
Myopia. The eyeball is too long, making it difficult to focus on distant objects. Onset age 5-11. Familial. 6% at age 6 years, and 16% at age 16 years.
Astigmatism. The cornea does not have a uniform curvature so that the image is distorted.

SQUINT (strabismus)
Definition. One eye is not directed at the object being looked at by the other.
Incidence. 3% of children will have a squint. Less than 1% are recognised by parents. Risk factors: family history of squint, difficult delivery, premature, neonatal jaundice, encephalitis or meningitis, cerebral palsy, mental retardation.
Clinically. When an ophthalmoscope is shone on to squinting eyes, the reflection of light is assymetrical. There is a latent squint if one eye stops looking at the light when covered (cover-uncover test). A paralytic squint is demonstrated by getting the child to look at a light as it is moved into all quadrants.

Aetiology.
1. Concomitant (non-paralytic) squint.
   - Idiopathic squints. Commonest. Usually convergent. 50% familial.
   - Severe hypermetropia. Excessive accommodation for near vision can cause excessive reflex convergence. Hypermetropia reduces as a child gets older.
   - Severe myopia may be associated with a divergent squint.
   - Unilateral refractive error.
   - Blindness in one eye.
   - Brain damage.
2. Incomitant (paralytic) squint: Paralysis of extraocular muscle(s).

Differential diagnosis.
- **A pseudo-squint** is an illusion caused by a wide nasal bridge or epicanthic folds.
- **A latent squint** is only evident when the squinting eye is covered or the child is tired or unwell. Rarely progresses to an overt squint or affects vision.
- **Alternating squint**: the eyes take up fixation alternately.
- **Incomitant (paralytic) squint**: The angle between the visual axes of the eyes varies depending on where the child is looking.
- **Concomitant (non-paralytic) squint**: The angle between the visual axes of the eyes remains constant wherever the child is looking.

Investigation. An amblyoscope is used to test older children for binocular vision (simultaneous perception, fusion and stereopsis).

Management. Refer any squint persisting after 6 weeks of age.
- Correct refractive errors. Patch the dominant eye for an hour a day to encourage the squint to alternate. Orthoptic exercises.
- Surgery to alter the balance of the extra-ocular muscles is most effective once a squint is alternating.

Prognosis. Uncorrected squints lead to reduced visual acuity (amblyopia). In extreme cases the weaker eye can be blind. Even if a squint is corrected in infancy full binocular vision may not develop.

VISUAL HANDICAP
Incidence. 25/100,000 children are registered blind (acuity < 6/60 in the best eye). 30/100,000 children are registered partially sighted (acuity < 6/24 in the best eye).

Risk factors. Familial blindness, congenital infection, prematurity, deafness, mental subnormality, cerebral palsy, hydrocephalus, epilepsy.

Aetiology.
1. Severe refractive errors (amblyopia).
2. Ocular pathology
   - Malformations: coloboma, no iris, small eye, no eye.
   - Corneal opacity.
   - Cataract: genetic, metabolic (galactosaemia), congenital rubella.
   - Glaucoma.
   - Retina: retrolental fibroplasia, inherited degenerations (retinitis pigmentosa), choroidoretinitis (toxoplasma, toxocara), retino-blastoma.
   - Trauma.
3. Optic nerve and tract:
   - Pituitary tumour.
   - Glioma.
   - Compresssion by bone overgrowth.
4. Cortical blindness

Management.
- Treat progressive disease.
- Spectacles for refractive errors.
- Special education.
- Aids including guide dogs.

Prognosis. Depends on the extent of associated handicaps and the response of the patient's family.

Glaucoma

Definition. Atrophy of the optic cup due to increased intraocular pressure. The growing eye is dilated by the pressure (buphthalmos).

Incidence. 3/100,000 children.

Aetiology.
- **Primary.** Malformation of the anterior chamber obstructs the outflow of the aqueous. Familial. Presents in infancy with buphthalmos.
- **Secondary** to uveitis, trauma, retinoblastoma, intraocular haemorrhage, Sturge-Weber syndrome, neurofibromatosis.

Clinically. Big eye. Hazy cornea (oedema) and conjunctivitis. Cupping of the optic disc. Older children may present with poor vision (reduced acuity and visual fields) and photophobia.

Investigation. Intraocular pressure by planometry. CT scan.

Treatment. Medical therapy may be used briefly in the interval between diagnosis and surgical decompression.

Cataract
Incidence. Uncommon.
Aetiology.
1. Congenital.
    • Rubella, cytomegalovirus infection.
    • Familial, usually autosomal dominant.
2. Acquired.
    • Perinatal hypoxia or hypoglycaemia.
    • Toxoplasmosis.
    • Metabolic: diabetes mellitus, homocystinuria, galactosaemia, hypocalcaemia, Cushing's syndrome or steroid therapy.
    • Syndromes: Marfan's, Down's.
    • Trauma.
    • Other eye diseases: retinoblastoma, anterior uveitis.
Clinically. Squint. White pupil reflex. Nystagmus.
Treatment. Cataracts which are mildly affecting vision should be left. Dense congenital cataracts must be excised by age 3 months to prevent amblyopia. After surgery infants need soft contact lenses and older children need spectacles. Intraocular lenses are contraindicated in children because the eye is still growing.
Prognosis. Depends on how long the cataract was present before extraction and any associated defects.

THE RED EYE
Aetiology.
• Trauma.
• Conjunctivitis: infection, allergy, dry eyes.
• Keratitis (cornea): herpetic ulceration.
• Scleritis and episcleritis.
• Anterior uveitis.
• Glaucoma.
• Cluster headaches.
History Sore or itchy? Precipitating trauma? Personal or family history of atopy?
Examination.
• Conjunctival injection that is more marked around the cornea suggests an intraocular problem or a corneal ulcer. Conjunctival injection that is greater towards the lids suggests conjunctivitis.
• Evert eyelids to look for foreign bodies, tears, pus.

- Visual acuity.
- Pupillary reaction to light and accommodation.
- Red reflex, fundoscopy.
- Stain cornea with fluoresceine to demonstrate ulcers.

Refer if conjunctival injection is most marked around the pupil (? a corneal or intraocular problem); if visual acuity is impaired; if the pupils react abnormally to light or accommodation; if there is corneal ulceration; if the fundus appears cloudy; if there is the suspicion of a penetrating eye injury.

Conjunctivitis
Aetiology.
Usually viral: enteroviruses, adenovirus, measles, herpes simplex, herpes zoster.
Commonly:
- Bacterial: S. aureus > Pneumococcus > Chlamydia. In Britain Chlamydia causes a mild disease caught in swimming pools, in tropical countries it causes blindness (trachoma). Ophthalmia neonatorum may be due to gonococcus or Chlamydia.
- Allergic: contact allergy, hayfever.
- Trauma or chemical irritation.
Occasionally:
- Dry eyes: exophthalmos, collagen vascular disease (JCA).
- Reiter's syndrome. Refer to ophthalmologist for steroid eye drops.
Investigation. Swab for bacterial culture and Chlamydia immuno-fluorescence.
Treatment.
- Viral: resolves spontaneously.
- Bacterial: antibiotic eye ointment.
- Allergic: cromoglycate eye drops.
- Ophthalmia neonatorum: systemic and topical antibiotics. Remember to treat both parents.

Retinoblastoma
Incidence. 1/20,000 live births. Age 0-3 years. 40% are autosomal dominant (all bilateral cases, 8% of unilateral cases).
Clinically. Squint. White pupil reflex. Poor vision. Painful red eye. Examine under general anaesthetic to confirm diagnosis.

Treatment. Small tumours can be burnt with a laser. The eye must be removed for large unilateral tumours. Bilateral tumours are irradiated. Chemotherapy for metastases.
Prognosis. 95% cure for small tumour. 100% mortality once metastasis has occurred.

EYELID PROBLEMS

Ptosis: drooping of the eyelid. Usually familial. Sometimes: damage to sympathetic nerves (Horner's syndrome) or the third nerve; thickening of the eyelid.

Stye: an infection of a lash follicle and associated sebaceous gland. S. aureus is the usual pathogen. Oral antibiotics if there is swelling of the lid. Hot flannels and removing the lash will encourage the stye to discharge. Antibiotic eye ointment prevents secondary conjunctivitis.

Chalazion: a granuloma within a tarsal oil gland (meibomian gland) presents as a tender swelling a few millimeters away from the lid margin. Treat as a stye. Any residual lump can be incised on the conjunctival surface.

Blepharitis: crusting of the lid margins. Three causes: seborrhoeic dermatitis; chronic infection (staphylococcal); contact dermatitis (cosmetics). Seborrhoeic and infective blepharitis respond to cleansing and antibiotic ointment applied to the lid margins. Allergic blepharitis responds to allergen avoidance and hydrocortisone cream.

Epiphora: a GP will see 1-2 infants each year with persistent watering of one or both eyes. Sometimes the discharge becomes purulent and pus can be squeezed out of the nasolacrimal duct. It is caused by obstruction of the duct which can be opened with a probe if it does not resolve by 4 months.

18. DERMATOLOGY

BIRTHMARKS

Pigmented naevus
Everyone has several. Arise as nests of melanin containing dermal and epidermal cells. May be seen at birth or only become evident as they grow. Deep naevi are blue, superficial naevi are brown. May be raised. Grow slowly. Occasionally become malignant, especially diffuse 'bathing trunk' hairy naevus.

Strawberry naevus (cavernous haemangioma)
Common. Becomes evident in the neonate. A raised, soft, red plaque. Gradually enlarges until 6 months of age then regresses to a flat or sunken pale scar by age 5-15 years. Massive naevi can cause thrombocytopenia, excessive local bone growth and cardiac failure.

Stork mark (capillary haemangioma)
Common. Flat pink mark at the nape of the neck and between the eyebrows. Fades by age 3.

Port-wine stain (capillary haemangioma)
Flat, purple-red, permanent. Usually an isolated lesion but may occur as part of the Sturge-Weber syndrome (port-wine stain in the trigeminal nerve distribution, intra-cerebral malformations, epilepsy, ipsilateral glaucoma, retinal dysplasia).

Spider naevus
Vessels radiating from a central arteriole. Most commonly on the face and upper body. Can be treated by coagulation (laser, heat, cryotherapy) but are best left alone. Multiple spider naevi are associated with cirrhosis and hereditary telangiectasia (Osler-Rendu-Weber disease).

NAPPY RASH

- Irritant dermatitis and intertrigo.
- Infections: impetigo, Candidiasis.
- Eczema.
- Seborrhoeic dermatitis.
- Psoriasis.

IRRITANT DERMATITIS
Incidence. Virtually every baby will have at least one episode.
Aetiology. Fæcal bacteria degrade urea in the urine to ammonia which burns the skin. Dermatitis is associated with infrequent nappy changes and plastic pants. Chronic irritant dermatitis suggests child neglect.
Clinically. A 'burn' in the nappy area, sparing the flexures. Secondary bacterial or candida infection is common. Sometimes secondary eczema develops outside the nappy area but disappears when the nappy rash settles.
Treatment. Prevent by frequent nappy changes, careful cleansing with baby lotion and routine use of a barrier cream such as zinc and castor oil. Leaving the baby out of nappies is an effective cure but the side effects can be messy. Severe cases are usually secondarily infected and a local antiseptic or antifungal cream may be needed.

CONTACT DERMATITIS
* Nappy rash. Indistinguishable from irritant dermatitis. Consider detergents and softeners used to clean towelling nappies.
* Medicated creams, clothing dyes, cosmetics, plants (hogweed). Once sensitized (1-2 weeks), a reaction develops 12-48 hours after exposure. Blisters and local oedema.

INTERTRIGO
Raw skin in body folds (genitocrural, perianal, axillae, neck folds). Obesity, neglect and nappies are risk factors. The skin is damaged by sweat, heat, friction and secondary infection. Use a topical antibiotic or antifungal if infected. Frequent drying and application of barrier cream to affected folds.

CANDIDIASIS
Common. Red patches on skin and white patches on mucosa, shallow ulcers with satellite lesions. Antifungal cream to skin and gel to oral lesions.

SEBORRHOEIC DERMATITIS
* **Young infants**. Common. Non-itchy, yellow-red greasy scales on the scalp (cradle cap), eyebrows, behind the ears, flexures, axillae, shoulders, napkin area. Hydrocortisone 1% cream if parents upset by this temporary imperfection. A keratolytic removes the cradle-cap (salicylic acid cream). Settles in late infancy.
* **Adolescents**. Common. Dandruff. Scaling affects the eyebrows, behind the ears, nasolabial folds, in the ears (otitis externa), chest, axilla, groins, perianal. Antifungals are more effective than steroid creams.

ATOPIC ECZEMA

Incidence. 3% of children. Starts by age 6 months in 75%, and by age 9 years in 90%. Improves by adolescence in 50%, and by age 20 in 80%.

Associated with:
- Family history of atopy (70%).
- Asthma and/or hayfever (50%).
- Urticaria.
- Food allergies.
- Dry skin (100%). 10% have icthyosis.
- Low itch threshold (itch after a change in mood or temperature).
- Dermographism.
- Alopecia areata and immune deficiency (rarely).

Clinically. Rash starts on face, and flexures (neck, elbow, wrist, knee) as a raw rash that oozes serum. Becomes thick and dry (hands, feet, flexures).

Complications.
- Skin infections (Herpes simplex, warts, S. aureus, fungi).
- Red man syndrome (whole body affected) is rare.

Investigations.
- IgE levels are elevated in the serum of 80%. Specific IgE to clinically recognised allergens is often detectable on RAST testing.
- Skin testing with suspected allergens.

Treatment.
- Only breast milk until 3 months old for infants at risk.
- Avoid allergens and non-specific irritants (soap, daily baths, wool, hot rooms).
- Wet eczema is treated with potassium permanganate soaks, topical antibacterials, and systemic antibacterials.
- Dry eczema. The following are listed in order of increasing strength and side effects: aqueous cream to skin; emulsifying ointment applied to the skin at frequent intervals, used instead of soap, and put in the bath water; steroid creams starting with hydrocortisone 0.5% and working up to fluorinated steroids (dermovate); coal-tar wraps; oral prednisolone.

PSORIASIS

Familial. Uncommon in childhood. A disease of white skins in cold countries. The basal epidermal cells multiply too quickly and cells are shed before they can form the protective layer of keratinised cells.

Clinically.
- Guttate psoriasis (gutta = drop): multiple, small, round, red, scaly patches. May follow streptococcal infection. Children > adults.

- Acute psoriasis: sterile pustules.
- Chronic psoriasis: non-itchy, red plaques with silvery scales. Punctate bleeding if scales are removed from a plaque. Nail pitting and separation from bed (onycholysis). Arthritis.

Investigation. Biopsy if appearance is atypical.

Treatment.

- In order of increasing strength: steroid creams; coal tar creams and dithranol; sunlight or sub-erythema doses of UVB; PUVA (psoralen + UVA), prednisolone; methotrexate; oral retinoic acid.
- Avoid precipitants: trauma (Köebner phenomenon), stress, lithium, chloroquine.

Prognosis. Guttate psoriasis lasts a few weeks but classical psoriasis may develop later. Classical psoriasis remits and relapses for life.

RING LESIONS

- Tinea.
- Impetigo.
- Herald patch of Pityriasis rosea.
- Nummular eczema.
- Psoriasis.
- Granuloma annulare

TINEA (Ringworm)

Incidence. Very common. Caused by various strains of Trichophyton, Epidermophyton and Microsporum fungi. Transmitted by contact with an infected person or animal.

Clinically. Itchy, scaly, red plaque which spreads with central clearing. On the head it appears as a bald patch with hairs broken off near the surface. On the feet the interdigital spaces become macerated and the nails can separate from their beds.

Investigation. Microscopy of skin scrapings treated with 20% potassium hydroxide to clear keratin debris. Fungal culture can help identify strain and the likely source of infection.

Treatment.

- Topical antifungal creams, shampoos and nail paints.
- Oral griseofulvin for 1-12 months.
- Oral imidazoles for severe infections resistant to other therapy.

IMPETIGO

Very common. Staphylococcus aureus > Streptococcus. Complicates any lesion that cracks the skin. Starts as a red spot that ulcerates and forms a yellow-brown crust. Spreads rapidly over the body. Very contagious. Isolate the child. Antibiotic cream to new lesions. Oral antibiotics for established lesions.

BUMPS IN THE SKIN

- Milia (neonates).
- Keratosis pilaris.
- Superficial urticaria.
- Acne.
- Molluscum contagiosum.
- Warts.
- Adenoma sebaceum (tuberous sclerosis).

MILIA (milk spots)

Very common during the neonatal period and last up to 3 months. Usually an isolated defect but occasionally associated with epidermolysis bullosa. Blocked pilosebaceous follicles. White papules the size of a pinhead on the face. No treatment. Differential diagnosis: Molluscum contagiosum, Adenoma sebaceum, infantile acne.

KERATOSIS PILARIS

Very common. Usually idiopathic, rarely associated with ichthyosis or vitamin B deficiency. Crops of minute horny bumps which block hair follicles on the limbs. Salicylic acid 2% in soft paraffin can be prescribed as a keratolytic in severe cases.

SUPERFICIAL URTICARIA

Pathophysiology. Dermal oedema in response to histamine:
- Often IgE mediated hypersensitivity to specific antigens (foods and drugs, candida and viral infections, nickel in contact with the skin).
- Sometimes a response to pressure (dermographism) or sunlight.
- Sometimes a pharmacological reaction (NSAID, tartrazine).

Clinically. Develops an itchy 'nettle rash' within 1 hour of exposure to the stimulus: red blotches, white wheals, blisters that may burst. Lasts a few hours after stimulus removed.

137

Investigation. Only for chronic or recurrent urticaria.
- Avoid allergen then challenge: elimination diets.
- Skin testing with a battery of antigens on patches.
- FBC for eosinophilia or signs of a reticulosis.
- Stool culture for parasites.
- ASOT (? streptococcal infection), viral titres.
- Autoantibodies (? collagen vascular disease)
- Serum immunoglobulins and cryoglobulins (cold urticaria).

Treatment.
- Avoid allergen.
- Oral antihistamine (H1 block) if allergen cannot be avoided.
- Cimetidine (H2 block) if antihistamine is inadequate.
- Prednisolone if antihistamines are inadequate.
- Hyposensitization is unreliable and dangerous.

Prognosis. 10% develop recurrent or chronic urticaria.

PAPULAR URTICARIA
Common. Caused by insect bites. A reaction in the epidermis and superficial dermis. Clusters of hard, itchy papules. Prescribe oral antihistamines.

ACNE
Incidence. Affects 25% of infants and 90% of teenagers. Boys > girls. Persists beyond age 25 in 15%.

Pathophysiology. Usually affects face and upper trunk.
- Hypersecretion of sebum causes greasy skin.
- Hyperkeratinisation in sebaceous glands blocks the outflow causing comedones (whiteheads and blackheads).
- Colonisation of the blocked sebaceous glands with the anaerobic diphtheroid Propionobacterium acnes which converts inactive lipid to long-chain fatty acids causing inflammatory papules.
- Secondary infection of papules causes pustules, cysts and scars.
- Psychological distress may be severe.

Acne is usually caused by normal levels of testosterone. Sometimes it is due to medication (contraceptive pills, prednisolone, phenytoin, barbiturates, phenytoin), irritants (cosmetics), endocrine abnormalities (Cushings, diabetes, virulizing tumour, polycystic ovaries).

Investigation. If a hormonal cause is suspected.

Treatment.
- Mild acne: keratolytic lotions (benzoyl peroxide) applied to face.
- Moderate acne: oral erythromycin.

- Moderate acne in adolescent girls: Dianette, which contains an anti-androgen (cyproterone acetate), is an alternative for adolescent girls who also require oral contraception.
- Severe acne: oral isotretinoin is a vitamin A analogue available only on hospital prescription. Causes dry skin and mucosae. 100% teratogenic.
- Scarring can be treated by dermabrasion.

Ultraviolet radiation and topical steroids are not of benefit.

MOLLUSCUM CONTAGIOSUM
Very common. Viral. Small pearly papules in clusters. Larger lesions may show a central dimple ('umbilicated'). Remove under local anaesthetic by cautery, freezing or pricking with phenol. Remit in a few months without treatment.

WARTS
Almost every child has warts and verrucae (warts on the soles of the feet) at some stage. Transmitted by direct contact or touching a wet surface contaminated by human papilloma virus. Genital warts suggest, but do not prove, sexual contact. Incubation period is 1-12 months. Last 3 months to 3 years until immunity develops. Painful verrucae or large warts should be treated with salicylic acid gel once nightly for six weeks. Resistant warts should be cauterized or frozen.

TUBEROUS SCLEROSIS
Rare. Autosomal dominant with variable penetrance and 80% new mutations.
- Ash-leaf macules are the first sign of the disease (95%).
- Adenoma sebaceum = small yellow or red papules on the nose, cheeks and chin (actually fibromas and not adenomas).
- Facial telangiectasia.
- A leathery patch of 'Shagreen skin' on the low back.
- Nodules beside the nails (periungual fibromata).
- White streak in the hair.
- Mental retardation (60%) and epilepsy (80%) due to disorganised areas of cerebral cortex that may be calcified.
- Tuberous malformations of other organs.

Prognosis. Die in middle age.

BUMPS UNDER THE SKIN

- Fat necrosis (neonates).
- Neurofibromas.
- Urticaria.
- Boils.

FAT NECROSIS
Seen in neonates after a traumatic delivery. Hard, subcutaneous nodules on head and limbs. Soften and disappear within a few months.

NEUROFIBROMAS
Neurofibromas are very common. They are localised proliferations of the Schwann cells and fibroblasts of peripheral nerve sheaths. Usually detected as asymptomatic subcutaneous nodules but may be tender if pressed.

Neurofibromatosis is a rare autosomal dominant characterised by:
- Multiple neurofibromas that may compress nerves and the spinal cord. Giant plexiform neuromas may become sarcomatous.
- Café aû lait spots are multiple (>5), large, ragged-edged, light brown and usually on the trunk.
- Mental retardation and epilepsy occur in 10% due to diffuse cortical dysgenesis.
- Bone cysts, skeletal deformities especially scoliosis.

Associated with (usually adults):
- Bilateral acoustic neuroma, gliomas, meningiomas.
- Phaeochromocytomas (1%).
- Orbital haemangiomas.
- Renal artery stenosis.
- Pulmonary fibrosis.

Treatment. Excision of symptomatic tumours.

DEEP URTICARIA (Angioedema)
Pathophysiology. Painful swelling of the dermal and subcutaneous tissues. Vasculitis with haemorrhage and infarction.

Aetiology. Localised or systemic excess of proteases over their inhibitors.
- Hereditary angioedema. Familial deficiency of C1-esterase inhibitor restricts the complement cascade. Minor trauma can cause massive swelling.
- Ischaemia or pressure.
- Any cause of superficial oedema.
- Erythema nodosum.

Clinically. Within 3 hours to 3 days of exposure to the stimulus a few large painful swellings develop.

Investigation. As for superficial oedema + C1-esterase inhibitor assay.

Treatment. Avoid precipitants.

- C1- esterase deficiency. Fresh frozen plasma for acute exacerbations. Danazol for prevention (induces C1- esterase inhibitor activity).
- Other causes. i.m. adrenaline + i.v. hydrocortisone + i.v. chlorpheniramine for acute episodes. Prednisolone or dapsone for prophylaxis.

Prognosis. Often recurrent.

BOILS

Common (1% of children each year). A localised infection of subcutaneous tissue by Staphylococcus aureus. Common in diabetes, immuno-incompetent children, and carriers of virulent strains of S. aureus. Check the urine for glucose and culture a swab from the boil. Prescribe a systemic antibiotic. If boils recur take a FBC and culture swabs from the nose axilla and groins.

ITCHY RASHES

- Scabies, lice, tinea, impetigo, Pityriasis versicolor.
- Eczema, urticaria.

SCABIES

Common. Spread by close contact. A mite (Sarcoptes scabiei) lays eggs in burrows under the skin. The larva hatches and emerges as the adult mite. After sensitization occurs (1-2 weeks) the child develops an itchy papulo-vesicular rash. Look for burrows on the wrists, interdigital spaces and axillary folds. Treat the child and family with gamma benzene hexachloride on two occasions 7-days apart. Clothing and bedding that has been in direct contact with skin can be decontaminated by washing in hot water.

LICE (Pediculosis)

- Head lice. Endemic. Girls > boys. Itchy head. Oval eggs (nits) attached to the hairs around the ears and the nape of the neck. Lice the size of a pin-head swing from hair to hair. Scratching results in impetigo. Treat the whole family with an insecticidal shampoo.
- Body lice. Uncommon. Epidemics associated with overcrowding. The louse lives in the seams of clothes. Erythematous papules where the louse has sucked blood. Insecticidal lotion to the body. Wash clothing in hot water.

PITYRIASIS VERSICOLOR
Fungal infection (Malassezia furfur). Small, light brown, scaly patches (pale against a dark skin). Moderately itchy. Microscopy of skin scrapings is diagnostic. Clears with antifungal cream.

KOEBNER PHENOMENON

Definition. Lesions appearing at the site of skin trauma.
Aetiology.
- Psoriasis.
- Eczema.
- Warts.
- Lichen planus
- Urticaria.

ERYTHRODERMA

Definition. Red skin over most of the body due to generalised skin disease.
Aetiology.
- Psoriasis.
- Eczema.
- Urticaria.
Complications.
- High output cardiac failure.
- Skin infection with bacteraemia.
- Hypoalbuminaemia due to protein loss from skin and gut.
- Impaired thermoregulation.

19. INFECTIONS

Infections characteristic of particular systems are discussed in the relevant chapters. For details see the 'Textbook of Paediatrics' by Forfar and Arneil.

NOTIFIABLE DISEASES

Acute encephalitis
Acute meningitis
Acute poliomyelitis
Anthrax
Cholera
Diphtheria
Dysentery
Food poisoning
Infective jaundice
Lassa fever
Leprosy

Leptospirosis
Malaria
Marburg disease
Measles
Mumps
Ophthalmia neonatorum
Paratyphoid fever
Plague
Rabies
Relapsing fever

Rubella
Scarlet fever
Smallpox
Tetanus
Tuberculosis
Typhoid fever
Typhus fever
Viral haemorrhagic
    fever
Whooping cough
Yellow fever

IMMUNISATION
Basic schedule:
- At 2 months, 3 months, and 4 months old:
    Diphtheria–tetanus–pertussis, polio, Haemophilus influenzae B.
- At 14 months old: Mumps–measles–rubella.
- At 4-5 years old: Diphtheria–tetanus, polio.
- At 10-14 years (girls only): Rubella.
- At 10-14 years (some health authorities): BCG.
- At 15-18 years: Tetanus and polio.

In 1993 more than 90% of eligible children had received all recommended immunisations.

Additional immunisations for children at special risk.
- BCG to Asian neonates.
- Hepatitis B to neonates born to carrier mothers.

Contraindications.
- General: Acute fever, severe local or systemic reaction to a previous dose of the same vaccine or a component of the vaccine.
- Live vaccine (MMR, BCG, oral polio): immunosuppressive drugs or systemic steroid therapy, pregnancy, immune deficiency syndromes (excluding HIV infection), lymphoreticular neoplasia.

143

But:

- A personal or family history of allergy is not a contraindication.
- A personal or family history of convulsions is not a contra-indication unless there is a progressive neurological disorder.
- Stable neurological conditions such as cerebral palsy or spina bifida are a positive indication for immunisation.
- Topical steroid therapy (inhaled or creams) is not a contra-indication.
- Immunisations can be done during an infection that does not cause a fever.
- Children with HIV infection can receive all vacines except BCG.
- Schoolchildren who have missed pre-school immunisations should be given catch-up doses.

FEVER

Definition. A fever is a rectal temperature above 38°C, an oral temperature above 37.8°C, an axillary temperature above 37.2°C.

Significance. 90% of children with bacteraemia have a rectal temperature of 39°C or more, however, only 5% of children with such a fever have a bacteraemia. Unless there is an obvious focus of infection a child should have an infection screen after 24 hours with a fever of 39°C or above. Between the ages of 6 months and 3 years a high fever may cause a febrile convulsion. Fever may actually help the body resist infection and a fever lower than 40°C cannot cause any damage unless the child becomes dehydrated or convulses.

Basic investigations. Urine culture, stool culture, FBC, CxR.

Differential diagnosis of fever.

Commonly:

- Exercise, emotion.
- Infection: respiratory>gastrointestinal>urinary tract.
- Overwrapping, hot room.
- Dehydration.

Occasionally:

- Neoplasia.
- Autoimmune disease.
- Thyrotoxicosis.
- Allergy or drug reaction.
- Large bruise, subdural haematoma, or tissue necrosis.
- Heart failure.
- A false fever can be recorded if the parents interfere with the thermometer or the child drinks a hot drink just before a thermometer is put in his mouth.

EXANTHEMATA
Erythema infectiosum
Parvovirus. Commonly causes small outbreaks among primary school children. Incubation 4-14 days. Bright red macular rash starts on the cheeks ('slapped cheek disease') and spreads to the body. The child is only slightly unwell.

Roseola infantum
Affects most children. Viral. 10-15 day incubation. The child is relatively well in view of the high fever which lasts for three days and fades as a maculopapular rash appears. Febrile convulsions are the only common complication.

Measles
Incidence. Commonest between age 5 months to 5 years. A GP will see 1-3 cases each year.
Clinically. 7-14 day incubation. Prodromal illness with high fever, snuffles, conjunctivitis, dry cough, Koplik spots, vomiting and diarrhoea. After 3 days a red macular rash starts on the head and spreads down. After another 3 days the child recovers and the rash clears leaving a brown stain. Infectious for 7 days after onset of rash.
Treatment. Children should be vaccinated at age 14 months. Non-immune contacts can be protected with measles vaccine or human immunoglobulin.
Complications. In the UK:
- Common: otitis media, bacterial conjunctivitis, febrile convulsions.
- Uncommon: secondary bacterial pneumonia, measles pneumonitis, post-infectious encephalomyelitis (1/1000).
- Rare: SSPE, death.

Rubella
Incidence. Endemic. In the UK 50-100 babies each year have congenital infection = 1/2000 live births. A primary maternal infection during the first trimester affects 40% of the fetuses (2% spontaneously aborted, 2% stillborn, 20% major malformation, 16% minor malformation). Maternal infection after the first trimester affects 5% of fetuses.
Clinically.
Post-natal infection. 2-3 week incubation. Little malaise or fever. Lymphadenopathy on the back of the neck. A faint, pink, macular rash. Infectious for 4 days after the onset of the rash. Unlike adults complications are rare in children (arthritis).

Congenital infection.
- Small for dates, failure to thrive.
- Rash, hepatitis, anaemia, thrombocytopenia, pneumonitis.
- Cataract, choroidoretinitis.
- Deafness.
- Pulmonary stenosis and patent ductus arteriosus.
- Mental retardation, microcephaly.

Treatment. Immunize children at age 14 months (MMR) or non-immune women before pregnancy.

HERPES VIRUSES
- Herpes simplex.
- Varicella zoster
- Epstein Barr virus
- Cytomegalovirus.

Herpes simplex
Virology. Transmitted by contact. Primary infection of skin and mucosa. Latent infection in local ganglion cells. Recurrent infection in skin. HSV1 (oral) and HSV2 (genital) cannot be distinguished antigenically.
Clinically.
- Gingivo-stomatitis. Incubation 1 week. Unwell young child with mouth ulcers (last 1 week).
- Cold sores. 30% of people have a recurrent blistering rash on the face for 10 days at a time. Alcohol applied to the blisters limits spread.
- Primary skin infection (herpetic whitlow).
- Conjunctivitis with corneal ulceration. Refer for slit-lamp examination and acyclovir eye ointment.
- Encephalitis is rare except in neonates who have acquired HSV2 from their mothers. 70% die and half the remainder are disabled.
- Generalised infection of immunosuppressed children.

Varicella zoster
- Chickenpox. Primary infection. Spread by droplet or vesicle fluid. 2-3 week incubation. Malaise, low fever. After 2 days develop oral and skin blisters. Complications: secondary infections of blisters causing scarring, encephalitis in pre-school children (1:10,000), primary pneumonia in adolescents.

- Recurrent infection (Shingles). Usually adults. Usually facial. Pain in a dermatome is followed by a blistering rash. Motor nerves may be affected. Oral or topical acyclovir may limit blistering if started within 72 hours of the first blister.

Infectious mononucleosis (Epstein Barr virus)
Clinically. Spread by droplet. Common in adolescence (kissing). Often asymptomatic. 4-7 week incubation. Prodromal illness: 3-7 days malaise, fever, nausea, headache. Main illness: 1-3 weeks tonsillitis, lymphadenopathy, hepatosplenomegaly. Common complications: persistent malaise, rash with ampicillin. Rare complications: neuritis and encephalitis (1%), airway blocked by pharyngeal oedema, immune haemolytic anaemia and thrombocytopenia.
Investigations. Lymphocytosis. Monospot for heterophile Abs.
Treatment. Prednisolone for airways ocdema.
Prognosis. 3/10,000 of those affected will die. Death is usually due to encephalitis or splenic rupture.

Cytomegalovirus
Incidence. Uncommon in childhood. Transmitted between adults by kissing and intercourse. A primary maternal infection during pregnancy (1/200 pregnancies) is more likely to infect the fetus than a reactivated infection. 1/2 of their newborn children excrete virus at birth. 1/2 of these infected neonates are clinically affected.
Clinically.
1. Usually asymptomatic. May mimic infectious mononucleosis.
2. Congenital infection.
- Malformations: microcephaly and cerebral palsy (20%), choroidoretinitis (10%), deafness (20%).
- Infected neonate: pneumonitis, hepatitis (60%), haemolytic anaemia and thrombocytopenic purpura (20%).
- Children with minimal brain dysfunction.
Treatment. Women at risk of sexually transmitted diseases should be counselled antenatally. Theraputic abortion after maternal infection would affect 3 normal babies for 1 abnormal baby.

MUMPS
Epidemiology. A paramyxovirus. Droplet spread. Infectious until 4 days after onset of illness. Endemic. Affects 60% of school children.

Clinically. 2-4 week incubation. Fever, headache, malaise. Parotiditis after 3 days. Complications: orchitis (20% of pubertal males), oophorotis, mastitis, deafness, meningitis.

Treatment. Vaccine. Prednisolone for bilateral orchitis.

HUMAN IMMUNE DEFICIENCY VIRUS (HIV)
See 'Haematology - Acquired Immune Deficiency Syndrome'.

MALARIA
Incidence. 220 children per year enter Britain infected by malaria. Most are born in this country of immigrant parents and contract malaria on holiday in India/Pakistan (Plasmodium vivax) or Africa (P. falciparum).

Clinically.
1. **P. vivax**. 2-9 week incubation. Fever, vomiting, diarrhoea, hepatospleno-megally.
2. **P. falciparum**. High fever, headache, jaundice, anaemia, hepatospleno-megally, haematuria. Cerebral malaria presents with vomiting, drowsiness and convulsions.

Management.
• Prophylactic anti-malarials, avoid mosquitoes.
• Identify the parasite on a blood film.
• Antimalarials and supportive care including blood transfusion.

TUBERCULOSIS
Incidence. In the UK 1% of children are tuberculin positive when tested in adolescence, 500 children are clinically affected each year (commoner in Asian children). A GP will see one affected child in a working lifetime. Children contract infection from adults with pulmonary TB. 70% of children have lung disease only, 24% had infections outside the lung only (usually lymph nodes), 6% had infections inside and outside the lung.

Clinically. Commonly limited to an asymptomatic primary focus in the lung with associated hilar lymphadenopathy. Spread is commoner in infants and young children. Pulmonary spread is associated with malaise, low fever and cough. Systemic spread is uncommon (meninges, bone, joints, kidneys, miliary TB).

Diagnosis. Tuberculin test (heaf test). Microscopy and culture of sputum or gastric washings.

Prevention.
- Slaughter of infected cattle and pasteurization of milk.
- Vaccination of at risk groups (Asian neonates, contacts of cases).
- Screening of at risk groups (doctors, immigrants).

Treatment.
- Asymptomatic with recent infection: isoniazid for 6 months.
- Symptomatic: isoniazid, ethambutol and rifampicin for 1 year.

Prognosis. Less than 1% of children with clinical TB will die.

STAPHYLOCOCCAL INFECTION

Epidemiology. S. aureus is the only common pathogen. Usually penicillin resistant. S. albus causes opportunistic infections (SBE).

Clinically.
- Asymptomatic infection (50% of children are nasal carriers).
- Skin: boils, styes, impetigo, paronychia.
- Food poisoning (toxic rather than infective).
- Pneumonia, septicaemia, meningitis, pseudomembranous entero-colitis.

STREPTOCOCCAL INFECTION

1. **Beta-haemolytic streptococci** (S. pyogenes) cause 5% of all childhood illnesses: respiratory tract including tonsillitis and otitis media, skin (impetigo and erysipelas).
    - Scarlet fever is caused by an erythrogenic toxin. It is a mild disease characterised by a rash of fine red macules on the limbs and trunk, a flushed face with pallor around the mouth, and a 'strawberry tongue'. The old skin may peel off as the rash fades.
    - The immune response to the streptococcus causes: post-streptococcal glomerulonephritis (see 'Kidney and urinary tract'), erythema nodosum, rheumatic fever and chorea (see 'Cardiovascular system').
2. **Alpha-haemolytic streptococci** (S. viridans) are weakly pathogenic: SBE.
3. **Non-haemolytic streptococci** (S. faecalis): UTIs complicating obstruction.

HAEMOPHILUS

Epidemiology. H. influenzae type B causes 99% of haemophilus infections in childhood. Affects 1 in every 600 children before their fifth birthday.

Clinically.

- 60% - Meningitis. Affected 700 children per year in the UK before mass immunisation started in 1992. Almost all under 3 years old. Of those affected, 10% were left with permanent neurological damage and 5% died.
- 15% - Acute epiglottitis.
- 10% - Septicaemia.
- 15% - Otitis media, pneumonia, sinusitis, septic arthritis, osteomyelitis.

Immunisation with Haemophilus influenzae B vaccine at 2 months, 3 months and 4 months of age induces protective antibodies in 95% of children.

NEISSERIA

- N. meningitidis (meningococcus). Usually causes an asymptomatic infection. Occasionally causes septicaemia and meningitis.
- N. gonorrhoea. Neonatal eye infection or sign of child sexual abuse.

20. GASTROINTESTINAL TRACT

ACUTE ABDOMINAL PAIN
Aetiology.
Common causes:
- Constipation.
- Gastroenteritis (3% of children per year).
- Appendicitis (4/1000 children per year).
- Mesenteric adenitis (4/1000 children per year).
- Urinary tract infection and hydronephrosis
- Emotional upset.

Less common causes:
- Torsion of the testis (3/10,000 boys/year).
- Intestinal obstruction and strangulated hernia.
- Trauma.
- Peptic ulcer, Meckel's diverticulum, oesophagitis.
- Pancreatitis, cholecystitis, hepatitis.
- Sickle cell anaemia, Henoch-Schönlein purpura.
- Pneumonia.
- Renal calculi.

Clinically. Older children complain of abdominal pain but infants can present with irritability, poor feeding, vomiting or diarrhoea.

Appendicitis
A disease of schoolchildren. Abdominal pain is followed by vomiting then fever. Tenderness localises to the right loin in 75%. Unlike mesenteric adenitis the pain and tenderness of appendicitis becomes gradually worse. Appendicectomy cures, but 1/1000 die.

Mesenteric adenitis
A disease of schoolchildren. Intermittent abdominal pain and mild tenderness develop during a febrile illness. Pain settles after a few days as the mesenteric lymph nodes shrink.

RECURRENT ABDOMINAL PAIN
Aetiology.
95% functional: infantile colic, recurrent abdominal pain of childhood.
5% organic: any cause of acute abdominal pain; migraine or periodic syndrome; food intolerance; epilepsy; cystic fibrosis; coeliac disease; Crohns; worms; lead poisoning; porphyria; diabetic acidosis.

Investigation.
- Blood for FBC, ESR, amylase, liver function tests; urine for sugar, protein, blood, microscopy and culture; stool for occult blood, microscopy and culture; abdominal X-ray, CxR.
- Refer for endoscopy or barium studies of the gut.

Infantile colic
15% of infants spend hours crying and pulling up their legs. This may be due to abdominal pain. Rarely lasts beyond 3 months of age. May settle on soya milk. A sedative is often more effective if given to the mother rather than the baby. Occasionally admission of the mother and child to hospital is necessary to break the cycle of anxious mother and crying baby.

Recurrent abdominal pain of childhood
10% of schoolchildren have recurrent abdominal pain. Incidence increases with age. Affects girls > boys after puberty. Not related to IQ or social class. More than half have a parent or sibling who was or is affected. Severity of pain reflects degree of stress. Consider parental disharmony, sexual abuse. 60% will suffer from non-organic pain in adult life.

VOMITING
Causes in the neonate
- Any cause of vomiting in infancy.
- Oesophageal atresia.
- Cerebral lesion (haemorrhage, hypoxia, infarct).
- Metabolic (kernicterus, hypoglycaemia).

Causes in the infant
- Normal possetting (regurgitation of small amounts of food mixed with ingested air a few minutes after a feed).
- Excessive regurgitation (flatulence, hiatus hernia, overfeeding).
- Any infection.
- Gastroenteritis.
- Food intolerance.
- Acute intestinal obstruction including pyloric stenosis.
- Coeliac disease.
- Any cause of abdominal pain including appendicitis.
- Whooping cough.
- Metabolic (uraemia, acidosis, congenital adrenal hyperplasia).
- Cerebral lesion.

Causes in the child
- Gastroenteritis.
- Any infection.
- Emotion.
- Any cause of abdominal pain.
- Metabolic (diabetic ketoacidosis, drugs, poisons).

Clinically. Bile or blood stained vomit and failure to thrive suggest serious pathology.

Hiatus hernia and gastro-oesophageal reflux
Common. Presents as an infant with normal weight gain despite excessive regurgitation. Diagnosis confirmed by barium meal. Reduce regurgitation by thickening milk feeds, nursing the baby upright after meals and giving domperidone. Resolves by age 1 year in 95%. A few require gastric surgery.

Oesophageal atresia
Incidence. 1/3000 live births. 90% are atresia with tracheo-oesophageal fistula (TOF) - the upper oesophagus ends after a few centimetres, the lower oesophagus opens into the trachea. 5% atresia without fistula. 5% fistula without atresia.

Clinically. Hydramnios (30%). Newborn dribbles and coughs. Milk enters lungs - chokes, becomes tachypnoeic and cyanosed. Soft nasogastric tube will not pass more than 10 cm.

Management. Confirm diagnosis by CxR after putting Gastro-graffin down a nasogastric tube. Nurse upright, put nasogastric tube on suction and arrange immediate surgical correction. 80% survive.

Pyloric stenosis
Incidence. 2/1000 live births. Boys (5:1). Familial.

Clinically. Vomiting starts 2 to 6 weeks after birth and becomes worse over a period of days or weeks. The vomiting becomes projectile but remains bile-free. The infant remains hungry. Visible gastric peristalsis is suggestive. Palpation of the thickened pylorus after a feed is diagnostic. Ultrasound can detect impalpable lesions.

Treatment. Ramstedt's operation = longitudinal incision of the pyloric muscle down to mucosa.

Gastroenteritis
Incidence. Each year 15% of infants present to their GP with gastroenteritis. Frequency declines from birth and levels off at 3% per year after age 5.

153

Aetiology.
Viral (40%) - Rotavirus, adenovirus, enteroviruses, hepatitis A.
Bacterial (20%) - E. coli, Salmonella, Shigella, Campylobacter.
Protozoa (5%) - Giardia lamblia, Entamoeba histolytica.
Unknown (35%).
Clinically. Vomiting often precedes diarrhoea. A moderate fever is common. Hospital admission is indicated for dysentery (bloody diarrhoea), dehydration (loss of >5% of body weight in an infant and >10% in an older child), or a severely toxic child.
Investigations. Investigate if diarrhoea lasts >3 days, or the child has been abroad recently, or the parents are food handlers, or there is an epidemic of bacterial infection. Stool for light microscopy, bacterial culture and electron microscopy. Urea and electrolytes. Refer to hospital if further investigations are needed.
Treatment. Oral rehydration with glucose-electrolyte solutions for 24 hours. Weigh daily until course of illness is evident. Anti-emetics and anti-diarrhoeal agents may be useful for older children with mild illnesses. Antibiotics may be indicated by the stool culture. A child who loses more than 5% of his body weight needs plasma electrolyte estimation, and may require i.v. fluids.

1. **Rotavirus.** Faecal-oral transmission. Commoner in winter. Usually affects infants and toddlers. Incubation 1-3 days. Presents as gastroenteritis. Virus is detected in stool by enzyme-linked immune globulin assay.

2. **Enteroviruses.** Coxsackie, ECHO (and rarely polio) viruses. Aerosol or faeco-oral spread. 5 day incubation. Cause: upper respiratory tract infections, herpangina, hand foot and mouth disease (Coxsackie A16), meningitis, encephalitis, myocarditis and post-viral fatigue syndrome.

3. **Hepatitis A.** Common and associated with overcrowding and poor hygeine. Faecal-oral transmission. Incubation 2-7 weeks. Often asymptomatic. Presents as fever, nausea and vomiting for a few days followed by diarrhoea, jaundice, tender hepatomegaly. Usually recover completely. Less than 5% develop chronic liver damage. Less than 1% die.

4. **Hepatitis B.** Uncommon. Spread by blood and secretions. Neonates are infected at or soon after delivery from a carrier mother. A purified antigen vaccine is available. Infection generally more severe than hepatitis A.

5. **Non-A, non-B hepatitis.** Similar to hepatitis B.

6. Salmonella

- **Salmonella food poisoning** is very common (more than 30,000 reported cases each year in the UK). Contaminated eggs and poultry. A few hours after infection the child develops colicy abdominal pain and vomiting followed by diarrhoea. The illness settles after a few days and antibiotics are not helpful.
- **Typhoid** affects 200 people each year in the UK (contracted abroad). Salmonella typhi is spread by faeco-oral contamination. The infection develops in the lymphoid follicles of the gut then becomes bacteraemic. Fever, cough, diarrhoea (may contain blood), vomiting, headache and confusion. Rash in 20% (Rose spots). Chloramphenicol or ampicillin. Vaccine is partially effective.
- **Paratyphoid** affects 100 people each year in the UK. It is milder than typhoid.

7. Shigella dysentery

3000 cases each year in the UK. Faeco-oral spread. Immunity does not follow infection. Shallow ulcers of the lower ileum and colon. Incubation 1-7 days. Diarrhoea (bloody), vomiting, abdominal pain, fever. Illness lasts 1-2 weeks. Treat with oral rehydration and ampicillin. Reactive arthritis is uncommon. Death is rare.

8. Cholera

2 imported cases each year in the UK. Faeco-oral spread. Incubation 1-3 days. Vomiting and profuse diarrhoea (rice-water stools) for 3 days. Tetracycline and insoluble sulphonamides help. 10% die. Vaccine is partially protective.

DIARRHOEA

Causes in the infant

- Normal (breast-fed babies pass up to 4 loose yellow stools daily).
- Starving (frequent small amounts of loose green stool).
  Diet (too much sugar or too much food).
- Gastroenteritis (15% of pre-school children and 3% of older children are affected each year). See chapter on 'Infections'.
  Necrotizing enterocolitis.
  Any infection.
  Obstruction (Hirschsprungs).
  Any cause of malabsorption.

Causes in the child

- Gastroenteritis.
- Any infection.
- Emotion.
- Toddler diarrhoea.
- Constipation with overflow.
- Any cause of malabsorption.
- Drugs especially antibiotics and laxatives.
- Inflammatory bowel disease is very rare in childhood. Crohns (1/100,000). Ulcerative colitis (4/100,000).

Toddler diarrhoea

Common. Reduced intestinal transit time results in frequent loose stools containing 'peas and carrots'. Microscopy and culture of stool is normal. The child is healthy and grows well. The condition resolves before school age.

MALABSORPTION

Fat (steatorrhoea)
- Cystic fibrosis (15%).
- Coeliac disease (35%).
- Other causes (15%): giardiasis, congenital intestinal malformations, Crohns, pancreatic insufficiency, biliary atresia, cirrhosis.

Carbohydrate
- Genetic.
- Secondary: gastroenteritis, coeliac disease.

Protein
- Any chronic diarrhoea.
- Enzyme deficiency (trypsinogen).
- Allergy (cows' milk).

Vitamins
- Any cause of steatorrhoea.
- B12 (Crohns).

Coeliac disease

Incidence. 1/1000 caucasian children in the UK. Does not affect black or oriental races.

Pathology. Gluten intolerance results in total villous atrophy.

Clinically. Usually presents as steatorrhoea, vomiting and failure to thrive when an infant is weaned. Mild forms may present later as iron deficiency anaemia, short stature, or delayed puberty.

Investigation. Duodenal mucosal biopsy shows recovery of villous atrophy on a gluten-free diet, and recurrence after a gluten challenge.
Treatment. Gluten-free diet for life. No barley, rye, wheat or oats.
Prognosis. Normal growth and good health on a strict diet. Associated with diabetes, thyroiditis, extrinsic allergic alveolitis and dermatitis herpetiformis. Less than 1% develop small bowel lymphoma.

Food intolerance

Incidence. 10% of children, 15% of atopic children, 1% of adults.
Aetiology.

- Food allergy affects 1% of children and 5% of atopic children. It is rare in adults. Type I hypersensitivity (histamine) - within minutes may develop eczema, urticaria, asthma, diarrhoea and vomiting, rhinitis, anaphylaxis). Type III (immune complex vasculitis) - within hours may develop deep urticaria, arthritis, nephritis, diarrhoea. Type IV hypersensitivity (T cell) - within days may develop necrosis. Common allergens include cows' milk, eggs, nuts, fish and shellfish, soft fruit, wheat.
- Enzyme deficiencies. Temporary lactase and sucrase deficiency after gastroenteritis causes diarrhoea. G6PDH deficiency causes haemolysis after eating broad beans.
- Pharmacological reactions are the commonest. Caffeine, flavourings (monosodium glutamate), amines (tyramine), preservatives (sodium benzoate), colourings (tartrazine), salicylates.
- Unknown mechanisms are involved in many drug reactions.

Clinically. Mild gastrointestinal symptoms are the commonest presentation. Milk allergy is more commonly suspected than proved.
Investigation. Elimination diet and challenge, jejunal biopsy, skin tests.
Treatment. Elimination diet, oral sodium cromoglycate for gut symptoms, oral antihistamines for urticaria, oral indomethacin for abdominal cramps and diarrhoea. Breast feed babies have a lower incidence of food allergy.

GASTROINTESTINAL BLEEDING

Haematemesis

- Mucosal tears secondary to vomiting are the only common cause of haematemesis (Mallory-Weiss syndrome).
- Swallowed blood (nosebleeds).
- Oesophagitis, peptic ulceration or gastritis.
- Oesophageal varices.
  Bleeding tendency (Henoch-Schönlein purpura, haemophilia).

Melaena or iron deficiency anaemia
- Any cause of intestinal obstruction.
- Any cause of haematemesis.
- Congenital malformations (Meckel's diverticulum).
- Intestinal infection.
- Rare causes (food allergy, intestinal telangiectasia or angioma, Crohn's).

Red blood in the stool
- Anal fissures are the only common cause of rectal bleeding.
- Rectal prolapse
- Any cause of haematemesis or melaena.

Investigation of gastrointestinal bleeding.
In most cases the blood loss is small and the diagnosis can be made clinically. In other cases consider: FBC, clotting screen, stool for microscopy and culture, sigmoidoscopy, gastroscopy, barium enema, colonoscopy, technetium scan (Meckel's), angiography.

Meckel's diverticulum
Incidence. 2% of children (10% develop symptoms). Male = Female.
Pathology. A remnant of the vitello-intestinal duct. Usually 2 feet proximal to the ileo-colic valve, 2 inches long. May contain ectopic pancreatic or gastric mucosa.
Clinically. Pain, melaena and anaemia (bleeding from ectopic gastric mucosa). Peritonitis (acute diverticulitis, impacted foreign body, or leak from a patent tip. If the tip is attached to the umbilicus (raspberry tumour) this can form the apex of a volvulus. Intestinal obstruction can follow invagination of the diverticulum especially if it acts as the focus for an intussusception.
Investigation. Locate the diverticulum by barium meal, radiolabelled technetium (concentrated by gastric mucosa), angiography.
Treatment. Excise.

Anal fissure
Fissures are usually caused by the passage of hard stools but consider self instrumentation, sexual abuse and inflammatory bowel disease. Increase dietary fibre and consider the short-term use of lignocaine gel, glycerine suppositories and a stool softener.

Rectal prolapse
Incidence. Common. Associated with constipation or diarrhoea.
Clinically. Mucosal prolapse reduces spontaneously. Full thickness prolapse is rare and suggests a weak pelvic floor (?spina bifida).

Treatment. Soften stools as described for anal fissure. Occasionally submucous phenol in arachis oil is used to stimulate fibrosis that anchors the mucosa. Circumferential perianal suture is seldom needed.

ACUTE INTESTINAL OBSTRUCTION
Aetiology.
Neonate:
- Congenital malformation of the gut. Duodenum (atresia). Small intestine (atresia, malrotation and volvulus, exomphalos and gastroschisis, polyp or cyst, hernia). Colon (Hirschsprungs). Anus (imperforate).
- Acquired intestinal obstruction (cystic fibrosis, necrotising enterocolitis, inspissated milk curds in premature babies).

Infant and young child:
- Intussusception, volvulus, strangulated hernia.

Older child and adolescent: strangulated hernia.

Clinically. Acute constipation (or failure to pass meconium within 48 hours of birth), bile-stained vomiting, abdominal distension and pain.

Investigation of suspected intestinal obstruction
- Plain abdominal X-ray for gas-dilated bowel and fluid levels.
- Barium enema if colonic obstruction is suspected.
- Barium meal if the obstruction may be proximal to the colon.
- Urea and electrolytes to assess hydration and exclude metabolic alkalosis secondary to fluid loss into the bowel lumen.

Hernia
- Diaphragmatic: respiratory distress, vomiting.
- Hiatus hernia: regurgitation, aspiration, anaemia.
- Umbilical, inguinal (indirect > direct), and femoral present with a lump, pain or intestinal obstruction. A congenital true umbilical hernia will usually resolve by age 2, otherwise all hernias require surgery to prevent obstruction and strangulation.

Mucoviscidosis (cystic fibrosis)
Incidence. 1/2000 live births. Autosomal recessive. The mucus secreted by exocrine glands is abnormally thick and sticky.
Clinically.
- 10% present with meconium ileus (15% of neonatal intestinal obstructions). A plug of meconium in the terminal ileum causes ischaemic ulceration and peritonitis.

- Pancreatic fibrosis - exocrine insufficiency - malabsorption.
- Obstructive jaundice and biliary cirrhosis are rare.
- 80% present with recurrent chest infections-. Bronchiectasis and cor pulmonale is the commonest cause of death in cystic fibrosis.
- Boys are azoospermic.

Management. A high sweat sodium is diagnostic.

Meconium ileus: laparotomy, enterotomy and lavage.

Subacute obstruction: oral N-acetyl cysteine.

Malabsorption: oral pancreatic enzyme supplements, protein-rich and fat-poor diet, salt supplements.

Chest: postural drainage and huffing, antibiotics for infections.

Intestinal atresia

Incidence. Duodenal atresia or stenosis occurs in 1/5000 live births (1/3 have Down's syndrome, other congenital abnormalities are common). Jejunal or ileal stenosis occurs in 1/5000 live births (commoner in cystic fibrosis). Colonic atresia occurs in 1/50,000 live births.

Clinically. Maternal polyhydramnios is common with proximal lesions (30% of duodenal atresias). Present with neonatal vomiting.

Treatment. Resection and reanastomosis. 80% survive.

Malrotation and volvulus neonatorum

Very rare. The caecum and mid-gut retain a narrow mesentery that can twist (volvulus) and strangulate. The base of this mesentery can form a band that obstructs the second part of the duodenum. Presents with vomiting a few days after delivery. Surgical correction.

Intussusception

Incidence. Commonest 3 - 12 months. Boys (2:1).

Pathology. Peristalsis pushes the terminal ileum into the distal colon and further unless treated. Ischaemia kills the invaginated bowel.

Clinically. Said to be preceded by a viral illness. Spasms of screaming and vomiting. Abdomen is distended and the intussusception may be palpable as a tender 'sausage'. Untreated the child becomes hot and shocked (dehydration). He may initially pass a normal stool but subsequently becomes constipated except for 'redcurrant jelly' stools (blood and mucus).

Management. In the first 24 hours a barium enema may confirm the diagnosis and reduce the intussusception but surgical correction is usually needed. About 5% recur.

Hirschsprung's disease
1/5000 live births. Familial. Boys (9:1). The bowel is narrowed for a variable distance proximal to the anus. The muscle of this bowel lacks autonomic ganglion cells. Usually presents as neonatal intestinal obstruction. Sometimes presents as chronic constipation, or failure to thrive, or enterocolitis. Rectal biopsy is diagnostic. Barium enema defines the extent of the lesion. A colostomy allows definitive surgery (anterior resection with reanastomosis to the anus) to be deferred until the child is bigger.

Imperforate anus
1/5000 births. The bowel may end above (40%) or below the levator ani (more likely to attain continence after surgery). 1/2 have a fistula to the vagina or bladder. 1/4 have other congenital abnormalities (heart, oesophageal or duodenal atresia). Present with acute intestinal obstruction on the day of birth. Diagnose by rectal examination. Plain abdominal X-ray with the child upside down - measure the distance from the colonic gas bubble to the anus.

CHRONIC CONSTIPATION
Aetiology usually reflects bad habits.
- Normal variation. A breast-fed baby may pass stools only once in 10 days.
- Lack of dietary fibre or inadequate fluid intake.
- Failure to develop a regular bowel habit (neglect by parents, stubborn child, mental retardation).
- Anatomical problem (painful anal fissure, anorectal stenosis and Hirschsprung's disease).
- Hypotonia (hypothyroidism, myopathy).
- Drugs and poisons (imipramine, lead).
Management. Empty bowel (oral senna, glycerine suppositories, phosphate enemas, manual removal under anaesthesia). Improve diet (adequate fibre and fluids including fruit juices). Lactulose for a few weeks. Regular toileting.

WORMS
- Threadworms are endemic in Britain.
- Whipworms, hookworms, tapeworms and larger roundworms are rare in Britain unless imported inside immigrants and holidaymakers.
- Toxocara canis and Toxocara cati are found in dog and cat faeces. 10% of urban children are or have been infested. Usually asymptomatic. Pre-school children may develop visceral larva migrans. Older children occasionally develop choroidoretinitis.

21. LIVER

JAUNDICE
A yellow colouration of the skin and mucosa due to the accumulation of excessive amounts of bilirubin. Racial pigmentation (melanin) and a dietary excess of carrots (carotine) and drugs (mepacrine) can also cause a yellow tint.

Pathophysiology.
- **Normal physiology.** Bilirubin is formed by the breakdown of haemoglobin. Hepatic Glucoronyl Transferase (GT) conjugates bilrubin with glucuronic acid. Conjugated bilirubin is water soluble and can be excreted in bile. Conjugated bilirubin is converted into urobilinogen by intestinal bacteria. Some urobilinogen is reabsorbed from the bowel and appears in the urine.
- **Haemolytic jaundice.** Excessive haemolysis results in overload of GT and jaundice with unconjugated bilirubin. If liver enzymes are defective, overload occurs with a normal degree of haemolysis. Unconjugated bilirubin in the skin can be converted to a water-soluble form by daylight. The water-soluble form is then excreted.
- **Obstructive jaundice.** If the biliary tree is obstructed conjugated bilirubin cannot pass into the bowel (pale stools) so it refluxes into the blood and is excreted in the urine (dark urine).
- **Hepatitis.** Hepatic enzyme insufficiency is complicated by intra-hepatic bile duct obstruction due to disruption of the normal liver architecture. The jaundice is due to conjugated and unconjugated bilirubin.

Jaundice after the neonatal period
Aetiology.
- **Hepatitis:** Usually hepatitis A (commonest cause of childhood jaundice in the UK), sometimes drug reactions. Occasionally: chronic active hepatitis, Reye's syndrome, galactosaemia.
- **Hepatic enzyme defect:** Gilbert's syndrome.
- **Increased haemolysis** (see 'Haemolytic anaemia').
- **Biliary obstruction:** Cystic fibrosis, congenital intra-hepatic biliary atresia, extra-hepatic biliary stenosis.
- **Cirrhosis.**
Investigation.
- Conjugated and unconjugated bilirubin, transaminase, alkaline phosphatase.
- Haemoglobin, blood film, reticulocyte count.
- Culture urine, blood and CSF.

- Viral titres (hepatitis A, hepatitis B, CMV, EBV, HIV).
- CxR.
- Hepatic ultrasound.
- Liver biopsy may show hepatitis or biliary atresia.
- Percutaneous cholangiography to localise extra-hepatic obstruction.

Obstructive jaundice
Clinically. Progressive jaundice and hepatosplenomegaly starting in the neonatal period.
Investigation. Hepatitis and biliary atresia cause similar biochemical disturbances but the former tends to cause a higher serum transaminase, unconjugated bilirubin and alpha-fetoprotein.
Treatment. Extra-hepatic obstruction may be resectable. Biliary atresia is progressive and the baby will die in infancy unless treated by liver transplantation.

Acute liver failure
Incidence. Rare in childhood.
Aetiology. Viral hepatitis; drugs (paracetamol); cirrhosis.

Cirrhosis
Aetiology.
- Hepatitis.
- Biliary obstruction.
- Metabolic (Wilson's disease, storage diseases).
- Venous congestion (cardiac failure, hepatic vein occlusion).

Clinically. Jaundice. Vomiting and confusion (metabolic encephalopathy). Haematemesis (oesophageal varices due to portal hypertension).

HEPATOMEGALY
In a child the upper border of the normal liver is level with the fourth or fifth intercostal space in the mid-clavicular line. The lower border is at the costal margin.
Aetiology. Hepatitis, tumour, storage diseases, venous congestion.
Differential diagnosis of hepatomegaly.
- Hepatomegaly.
- Prominent Reidle's lobe of the liver.
- Hyperinflation of the lungs.

22. KIDNEY AND URINARY TRACT

URINARY TRACT INFECTION (UTI)

Definitions.

Significant bacteriuria = more than 100,000 organisms per millilitre of urine, with the same species and serotype being isolated from repeated clean catch specimens. If urine is obtained by suprapubic aspiration 10,000 organisms per millilitre is diagnostic.

UTI = significant bacteriuria and symptoms of urinary infection.

Incidence.

- 5% of children have at least one UTI. A GP would see one new case every couple of years. 3% of schoolgirls and 1% of schoolboys have at least one UTI. There are no geographical, social or ethnic variations.
- 2% of infants have asymptomatic bacteriuria (commoner in males). The incidence falls rapidly after the neonatal period, is stable during the school years, and becomes more common as sexual activity starts. The prevalence of asymptomatic bacteriuria is 2% in schoolgirls and 0.04% in schoolboys.
- 66% of children presenting with the symptoms of a UTI have sterile urine.

Bacteriology.

Neonates: 75% E. coli, 11% Klebsiella, 14% others.

Children: 85% E. coli, 6% Proteus, 3% S. albus.

Risk factors.

Structural or functional abnormalities are found in 45% of children presenting with UTI (90% under the age of 2 years, 60% under 5).

- 33% Vesico-ureteric reflux (VUR) prevents the bladder from emptying completely. The higher the reflux reaches up the ureter, the commoner is chronic pyelonephritis. Functional VUR is often familial and affects 1/3 of siblings of the index case, it tends to improve with age. VUR is sometimes due to malformation.
- 4% Stone or obstruction. Pelviureteric junction obstruction, ureteral stricture, cystoureteric junction obstruction, neurogenic bladder (spina bifida). Boys may have urethral valves and urethral or meatal stenosis.
- 5% Renal malformation (duplex or polycystic kidneys).
- Diabetes mellitus.
- Sexual abuse.

Clinically. Obstruction is suggested by a mass (enlarged bladder or kidney), hypertension and dehydration.

- Neonates. Irritability and sluggishness, tachypnoea and apnoea, hypertonia and convulsions, shock and jaundice. 50% have bacteraemia. Fever is uncommon.
- Age 1 month to 2 years. Smelly urine. Irritable and tearful. Vomiting, feeding problems and failure to thrive.

- Age 2 to 5 years. Abdominal pain, fever, dysuria, frequency. 40% of children with daytime enuresis and 10% with bedwetting have bacteriuria.
- School age. Increasingly like an adult. Enuresis, dysuria, frequency haematuria and loin pain. Fever is less common.

Investigations.

To confirm the diagnosis - obtain urine. Suprapubic aspiration from a sick infant. A 'clean catch' specimen is less often contaminated than an adhesive bag urine and less traumatic than sterile catheterisation. A mid-stream urine (MSU) if continent.

- Urine analysis by indicator sticks. In 95% of infections the urine will be positive for, one or more of, blood, protein, nitrites and leucocytes.
- Urine microscopy for white cells (>10 per microlitre), bacteria and casts.
- Urine culture to confirm diagnosis and define antibiotic sensitivities.

Consider: serum creatinine, bilirubin, FBC (anaemia, leucocytosis).

Every child should be investigated during or after their first UTI:

- Ultrasound scan (USS) for renal scars of chronic pyelonephritis (CPN) and urinary tract dilatation (reflux or obstruction)
- Plain abdominal X-ray for stones and spina bifida.

Further investigations once urine is sterile:

- DMSA scan (^{99}Tc dimercaptosuccinic acid scintigraphy) identifies 80% of CPN scars.
- IVU if the less invasive DMSA scan is not available.
- DTPA scan (^{99}Tc diethlenetriaminepenta-acetic acid scintigraphy) to assess obstruction and measure renal function.
- Micturating cystourethrogram (MCU) to assess reflux.

Age 1: DMSA or IVU, and DTPA or MCU

Age 1 to 7: DMSA scan or IVU. DTPA or MCU if other tests abnormal.

Age 7+: IVU and DMSA scan after recurrent infections only.

Treatment. Treating asymptomatic bacteriuria with no evidence of CPN, may eliminate an avirulent strain allowing re-infection with a virulent strain.

- Acute UTI. Trimethoprim at full dose for 7 days then low dose until investigations completed. Alternative antibiotics include co-trimoxazole, nitrofurantoin and cephalosporins.
- Prevention. Prophylactic trimethoprim and regular urine cultures until 7 years old if there is VUR, CPN, recurrent infections, or anatomical abnormality. Surgery for stone, obstruction, severe VUR.

Prognosis. 50% of uncomplicated UTIs and a higher proportion of complicated cases recur in childhood. Pyelonephritis in childhood is associated with a 10% risk of chronic renal failure in adult life.

CHRONIC PYELONEPHRITIS
Commonest cause of hypertension and renal insufficiency in children and young adults. 95% follow UTI with intra-renal reflux in childhood.

DIFFERENTIAL DIAGNOSIS OF RED URINE
• Haematuria (whole red cells) or haemoglobinuria (free haemoglobin).
• Myoglobinuria: muscle trauma, 'march' haematuria in adolescents, post-infectious.
• Foods and drugs: beetroot, blackberries, nitrofurantoin.
• Other: porphyrins, urates.
Investigation: urine analysis for haemoglobin. Urine microscopy.

DIFFERENTIAL DIAGNOSIS OF HAEMATURIA
• Urinary tract infection.
• Glomerulonephritis.
• Tumour: nephroblastoma, renal angioma, polycystic disease.
• Obstruction or urinary stones.
• Other less common causes: bleeding tendencies, drugs (cytotoxics), trauma and foreign body, renal infarction (?SBE).
Investigation. urine microscopy and culture, ultrasound scan, abdominal X-ray, coagulation studies, red cell and platelet counts, renal biopsy.

ACUTE RENAL FAILURE
The sudden inability of the kidneys to maintain body haemostasis due to a reduced GFR. Results in salt and water retention (oliguria, oedema, hypertension, heart failure), retention of waste products (urea, creatinine) and metabolic acidosis (vomiting and acidotic respiration). Urine is very concentrated in pre-renal failure and very dilute in intrinsic renal failure.
Aetiology. Common causes include post-operative hypovolaemia (35%), haemolytic-uraemic syndrome (25%), acute tubular necrosis (15%), glomerulonephritis (10%).
Classification.
• Pre-renal failure (reduced renal artery blood flow): usually due to hypotension. Occasionally due to renal artery/arteriole occlusion, renal vein thrombosis (fetal or neonatal).
• Intrinsic renal failure: acute tubular necrosis (usually secondary to pre-renal failure or drugs), papillary necrosis, glomerulonephritis, interstitial nephritis, haemolytic-uraemic syndrome.
• Post-renal (obstruction in the tubules or urinary tract): usually associated with spina bifida.

Management.
- Investigate and treat the cause.
- Reduce fluid overload: restrict fluid intake, intravenous frusemide.
- Reduce hyperkalaemia and acidosis.
- Feed: provide adequate calories (150 kcal/kg) as carbohydrates. Limit protein (1 g/kg body weight).
- Treat hypertension.
- Dialysis.

Prognosis. depends on aetiology. About 50% die.

CHRONIC RENAL FAILURE (CRF)

The progressive and irreversible loss of renal function.

Incidence. A GP will see a child with CRF every 100 years.

Aetiology.
- Chronic pyelonephritis.
- Chronic glomerulonephritis.
- Congenital renal abnormalities.
- Familial diseases.

Clinically. Polyuria, polydipsia, secondary enuresis, anaemia, failure to thrive, hypertension.

Investigation. Dilute urine which may contain casts. Serum: raised creatinine, low sodium, high potassium, metabolic acidosis.

Management. Treat hypertension and UTIs vigorously.
- Diet: high calorie diet, low protein, low potassium.
- Prevent renal osteodystrophy by giving hydroxylated vitamin D supplements, restricting dietary phosphate, and prescribing calcium carbonate to bind phosphate in the gut.
- Salt supplements if hypovolaemic from polyuria.
- Sodium bicarbonate supplements if acidotic.
- Hyperkalaemia: give calcium resonium.
- Dialysis: continuous ambulatory peritoneal dialysis (CAPD), haemodialysis (home or hospital ?).
- Transplantation.
- Support the child and the family.

Prognosis. Home haemodialysis 85% survival at 5 years. Hospital haemodialysis 66% survival at 5 years. CAPD 85% survival at 1 year. Transplantation 75% survival at 4 years.

NEPHROTIC SYNDROME

Proteinuria causing hypoalbuminaemia and oedema.

Aetiology.
- 90% Glomerulonephritis (usually 'minimal change glomerulopathy').
- 20% Secondary to Henoch-Schönlein syndrome, SLE etc.

Clinically. Oedema and ascites. Muscle wasting.

Investigations.
- 24 hour urine protein >1 g.
- Serum albumin is <25 g/l.
- Percutaneous renal biopsy in severe cases.

Treatment.
- High protein, low salt diet. Moderate fluid restriction.
- Diuretics.
- Prednisolone for 4 weeks, repeated for recurrences.
- Cyclophosphamide for frequent recurrences.

Prognosis. Most remit after a few years.

CONGENITAL ABNORMALITIES

Bilateral renal agenesis
Always rapidly fatal. 4/1000 stillbirths and early neonatal deaths. Males (2:1). Oligohydramnios. 'Potter facies' = low set ears, wide set eyes, flat nose, small jaw. Commonly associated with bilateral pulmonary hypoplasia. Diagnosis confirmed by ultrasound.

Unilateral renal agenesis
1/1000 live births. More common in boys. Frequently have ipsilateral absence of ureter and abnormal external ear. Contralateral kidney hypertrophies and renal function is normal.

Renal hypoplasia and dysplasia
Hypoplasia is usually associated with dysplasia (masses of undifferentiated mesenchyme that can form cartilage and smooth muscle). The affected kidney is small and cystic but the dysplasic tissue may be so big as to obstruct delivery. Increased incidence of UTI, chronic pyelonephritis, and hypertension.

Ectopic kidneys
The kidneys form in the pelvis as discs with the ureter arising anteriorly. Ectopic kidneys retain this appearance. Usually in the pelvis but may be anywhere in the abdomen, even fused with the normal kidney. Ureter may open into the bladder, urethra or vagina. Initial function is usually normal. Prone to UTI, obstruction and reflux.

Horseshoe kidneys
Normal lumbar kidneys fused at their lower poles. Ureters arise anteriorly.

Pelviureteric junction obstruction
Boys > girls. Hydronephrosis of fetal kidney on antenatal ultrasound. Infant or child with hydronephrosis (loin mass, UTI, hypertension). Diagnosis confirmed by ultrasound scan or DTPA scan with frusemide in mild cases. Treated by nephrostomy then pyeloplasty or nephrectomy.

Vesicoureteric junction obstruction
May be functional, anatomical. Presents with UTI. Usually cured by reimplanting the ureters at another site in the bladder.

RENAL CYSTS
Simple cysts
Usually single, usually unilateral and only cause problems if large.

Infantile polycystic disease
Autosomal recessive. Cysts extend radially from renal medulla to cortex. Antenatal diagnosis by ultrasound at 16 weeks gestation. Cysts may obstruct delivery. A few die as neonates. Usually presents in infancy or early childhood with bilateral renal masses, renal failure and hypertension. Hepatic cysts and fibrosis cause portal hypertension.

Adult polycystic disease
Autosomal dominant. Usually presents in adults but may start in childhood. Spherical cysts scattered throughout kidneys and liver. Hypertension in childhood and progressive renal failure as adults.

Juvenile nephronophthisis
Autosomal recessive. Renal medullary cysts. Progressive renal failure in late childhood.

Differential diagnosis of a renal mass.
Hydronephrosis.
Dysplastic kidney.
Compensatory renal hypertrophy (contralateral kidney hypoplastic).
Simple renal cyst.
Polycystic disease of the kidneys.
Tumour (neuroblastoma, renal).

RENAL TUMOURS

- Primary malignant: mostly nephroblastomas; occasionally fibrosarcomas, teratomas, adenocarcinomas.
- Primary benign (uncommon).
- Secondaries (uncommon and asymptomatic).

Nephroblastoma (Wilm's Tumour)

Incidence. 1/10,000 live births. Presents by age 5 (usually 2-4).

Pathology. Starts before or soon after birth as a mass of embryonic renal tissue with mesenchymal and epithelial elements. Varies from undifferentiated to highly differentiated (mesenchyme - muscle, osteoid, cartilage; epithelium - glomeruli, tubules). Forms a large grey mass that infiltrates surrounding tissues. 10% bilateral. At diagnosis 25% have metastasized by blood to lungs, liver, vertebrae.

Clinically. Presents with mass (50%), hypertension (60%), abdominal pain (30%), haematuria (10%). Sometimes fever, polycythaemia (erythropoetin).

Investigations. As for UTI. Bone scan and CxR for metastases. Needle biopsy is contraindicated (haemorrhage and tumour spread).

Treatment. Nephrectomy then radiotherapy and actinomycin D.

Prognosis. 50-90% total cure depending on tumour differentiation, size and spread.

23. GENITALS

GROIN LUMPS
- Hernia (congenital indirect inguinal > femoral).
- Lymph node.
- Testis.
- Rarely: hydrocele of the cord, lipoma, aneurysm.

Undescended testis
Incidence. Undescended testes are found in 100% of premature male neonates of 32 weeks gestation, 5% of boys at full term, and 0.5% of boys at 1 year. Spontaneous descent is rare after infancy. In 25% of cases both testes are undescended.
Pathology. Aetiology is unknown. An 'undescended testis' lies along the line of descent of the normal testis, often near the external inguinal ring. The testis is usually smaller than average. If the testis is not in the scrotum by age 4 the spermatic tubules and germ cells atrophy.
Differential diagnosis of empty scrotum.
- Undescended testis.
- Retractile testis. Can usually be coaxed down into the scrotum if the child is in a warm room with hips flexed and abducted.
- An 'ectopic testis' lies away from the normal line of descent, and is often palpable in the superficial inguinal pouch.
- Atrophic testis (unrecognized torsion, mumps, Klinefelter's syndrome, Kalman's syndrome, Noonan's syndrome).
- Various causes of ambiguous genitalia including absent testis (agenesis or infarction during fetal growth).
Clinically. An undescended testis is usually impalpable. The ipsilateral scrotum is poorly developed.
Investigations. Ultrasound scan to locate the testis. Laparoscopy if the ultrasound is negative. IVP for associated renal anomalies. Karyotype and electrolytes if both testes are undescended.
Treatment. Human chorionic gonadotrophin therapy causes testicular descent in 30% of cases of bilateral cryptorchism and 15% of unilateral cases. Surgery between age 2 and 4 is more successful in preserving fertility.
Prognosis. A school child with undescended testes will be teased.
Malignant tumours develop in 0.3/1000 scrotal testes, 10/1000 undescended testes found in the groin, and 50/1000 of those found in the abdomen.
30% of those with unilateral undescended testes are sub-fertile, and 60% of those with bilateral undescended testes are infertile.

- Following orchidopexy some testes atrophy and hormone replacement may be needed in adolescence.
- Torsion is more common in undescended testes.

SCROTAL PAIN
- Torsion of the testis.
- Trauma.
- Strangulated inguinal hernia.
- Testicular neoplasm.
- Haematoma due to a bleeding tendency.
- Referred pain.

Torsion of the testis
Commonest between age 10 and 25. Also common during infancy.

Pathology. The spermatic cord can twist if it is not attached to the testis in the usual manner. Less commonly, the testis can twist if it is attached to the epididymis by an unusually long mesentery. Either rotation compromises the testicular artery that runs down the spermatic cord and through the epididymis. The testis then infarcts within 4 hours. The associated acute hydrocele contains blood.

Clinically. Sudden onset of severe pain in the lower abdomen and testis. Vomiting is common but fever is not. Usually no precipitating trauma or exertion. The affected testis is tender, high, and often horizontal.

Management. Unless there is a definite history of mumps, UTI or trauma an acutely painful scrotum should be immediately explored surgically. The torsion is untwisted and both testes are fixed to prevent rotation.

SCROTAL SWELLINGS
1. Primary scrotal swelling:
   - Varicocele
   - Cystic: a cyst of the epididymis (distinct from the testis), a hydrocele or haematoma (enclose or obscure the testis).
   - Solid and cold: testicular tumour, tuberculous epididymitis.
   - Solid and hot: orchitis (mumps), torsion, acute epididymitis.
2. Extends down from the groin:
   - Inguinal hernia.

Varicocele
Incidence. 5% of adolescents. Usually (19/20) on left side.
Pathology. Dilatation of the pampiniform plexus which drains through the testicular vein to the inferior vena cava on the right and the renal vein on the left. Rarely (4/1000) due to a hypernephroma growing into the left renal vein.
Clinically. A varicocele feels like a bag of worms which shrinks when the patient is lying down. A large varicocele may ache. The ipsilateral testis may be smaller. Relative infertility.
Management. Ligation is indicated for pain or infertility.

Hydrocele
The testis sits on the tunica vaginalis like a tennis ball on a glove. A hydrocele is like a glove filled with fluid. Fluid collects because of:
- Connection with the peritoneal cavity. The congenital hydrocele is a soft translucent swelling surrounding the testis. It can be emptied by elevation. Usually vanishes during infancy.
- Failure of absorption of fluid by the tunica. The primary 'infantile' hydrocele extends a variable distance up the cord.
- Overproduction of fluid (due to infection, trauma, tumour, torsion).
- Block of lymphatics (due to infection, surgery).
- Systemic oedema.

Management. No investigation is indicated if the testis is palpably normal and the hydrocele developed in infancy. Refer for surgery if it persists into childhood. The management of an abnormal or impalpable testis is described under 'testicular tumour'.

BALANITIS
Inflammation under the foreskin is common in young boys. Caused by chemical irritation (nappy rash) or pyogenic organisms. It causes pain, dysuria and a purulent discharge. Treat with washing and systemic antibiotics.

CIRCUMCISION
Excision of the foreskin.
Indications: recurrent balanitis and phimosis, religious beliefs.

VULVOVAGINITIS
Incidence. Common.
Clinically. Perineal irritation. Dysuria. Discharge.
Investigation. Swab for bacteriology and mycology. Urine culture. Sellotape test for threadworm eggs.

Differential diagnosis.
- Chemical irritation (ammonia from urine breakdown on nappy).
- Mechanical irritation (masturbation).
- Intertrigo.
- Thrush.
- Threadworms.
- Streptococcal and Staphylococcal infections.
- Sexually transmitted diseases (sexually abused children or sexually active adolescents).
- Other causes of vaginal discharge, including that caused by a foreign body.
- Eczema, psoriasis.

Treatment. Be aware that the parents may have strange ideas about the cause and prognosis of the condition. If there is no specific cause advise regular washing without soap, careful drying, and cotton pants. Barrier creams containing an anti-fungal and antiseptic are useful. An oestrogen cream may succeed when all else fails.

AMBIGUOUS GENITALIA (INTERSEX)
Ambiguous genitalia may be obvious at birth. A disorder of sex differentiation may present as a female with clitoral enlargement, inguinal masses or herniae. Males with hypospadias, cryptorchidism or micropenis should also be investigated.

Clinical assessment.
- The child. If a gonad can be felt the child is probably male.
- Mother. Is there a source of excessive androgens.
- Examine siblings, father and relatives.

Investigations.
- Urgent electrolytes to exclude salt loosing congenital adrenal hyperplasia.
- 17 hydroxyprogesterone levels are high in CAH.
- LH and testosterone levels are extremely high with androgen insensitivity.
- Karyotype.
- Ultrasound. If a uterus is present there will not be any functioning testicular tissue. The ultrasound may demonstrate impalpable gonads if there are any present.
- Laparoscopy to biopsy of any gonads found on ultrasound.

Gender assignment. Karyotype is not decisive. Functionally normal external genitalia are the highest priority. If a uterus and ovaries are present then pregnancy may eventually be possible either normally or by in vitro fertilisation and embryo transfer.

- A neonate with ambiguous genitalia should not be named (or registered) until the sex has been 'chosen'.
- In general, virulised females should be surgically or hormonally feminised.
- Partially masculinised males who show phallic growth in response to testosterone should be masculinised. Non-responders and cases of testicular feminisation are better as females.
- After the newborn period the child should, in general, continue to be raised according to the assumed gender.
- Intra-abdominal gonads should be removed to avoid the risk of malignant change.
- The appropriate hormones should be given to initiate and maintain puberty.
- The family will need long term supportive counselling.

Virulised females (46XX)
Fetal exposure to androgens in the first trimester causes labioscrotal fusion with normal female internal genitalia. Later exposure simply causes clitoral hypertrophy. Aetiology:
- Fetal androgens. CAH is the commonest cause of virulisation.
- Intra-uterine exposure to maternal androgens: progestogens taken by the mother; adrenal or ovarian tumour in the mother.
- Part of a dysmorphic syndrome.
- Idiopathic.

Inadequately masculinised males (46XY)
Mild cases present as a male with hypospadias or cryptorchidism. Extreme cases = 'testicular feminisation'.
- Inadequate testosterone (gonadal dysgenesis, enzyme defects, pituitary failure).
- End-organ resistance to androgens is due to defective activation of testosterone in target tissues (5 alpha reductase deficiency), or androgen receptor defects. Born as 'females' but the vagina is short and there is no uterus. The testes are often in the labia. Some masculinisation may occur at puberty.

Hypospadias
Incidence. 1/350 boys.
Pathology. The penis forms as an ectodermal outgrowth with an endodermal plate on its inferior surface. The borders of the ectodermal outgrowth curve inferiorly, rolling the endodermal plate into a tube (urethra), and fuse in the midline. The penile urethra so formed opens at the base of the glans. Then the

terminal part of the penile urethra develops as an ingrowth of the surface epithelium.

- Mild hypospadias: the terminal part of the urethra does not form, and there is a 'hooded' prepuce.
- Moderate hypospadias: the urethra opens on the ventral surface of the penis at some point between the scrotum and glans. The corpora spongiosum and cavernosum do not form distal to the urethral opening. The penis curves ventrally.
- Severe hypospadias. The urethra opens between the scrotal folds, the testes do not descend. ? Intersex.

Investigations: karyotype, IVU, micturating cysto-urethrogram.
Management. The foreskin is used to fashion the distal urethra. In mild and moderate forms urinary and sexual function can develop normally after surgery.

Epispadias
The urethra opens on the dorsal surface of the penis. Surgery at age 3-4 years allows a variable degree of continence.

True hermaphrodites
Very rare. There is well developed ovarian and testicular tissue in the same or opposite gonads. The internal organs develop according to the nature of the ipsilateral gonad. The external genitalia are ambiguous. Breast development and virilisation are common at puberty. 50% menstruate at puberty. Karyotype is 60% 46XX, 10% 46XY, and 30% 46XX/46XY.

Gonadal dysgenesis
3/10,000 live births. Karyotype is usually 46XY (males with normal external genitalia but no testicular tissue). Sometimes 45X0 (Turner's syndrome = females without ovaries).

24. ORTHOPAEDICS

LIMB PAINS
- Psychological 'growing pains".
- Any febrile illness can cause limb pains.
- Trauma to soft tissues, bones and joints (acute trauma, overuse, non-accidental injury).
- Other diseases affecting soft tissues, bones, and joints.

Psychological 'growing pains'
Incidence. Affect up to 10% of children at any time. Peak incidence at age 11 when 30% of girls and 20% of boys are affected.
Clinically. Pain usually in bones not joints. Pains are related to emotional stress. During an attack there are no physical signs. The child is well for days or weeks between pains. Recurrent headaches and recurrent abdominal pains occur in at least one third.
Prognosis. Often converts to migraine in adult life.

BONE PAINS
- Fracture: acute and repetitive strain.
- Osteomyelitis.
- Infarction: Sickle-cell anaemia.
- Bone tumours.
- Metabolic disorders: rickets, scurvy.

Osteomyelitis
Incidence. Commonest in infants. Boys > girls. 75% S. aureus. Salmonella in sickle cell disease. Infection usually follows bacteraemia, but sometimes follows penetrating trauma.
Clinically. Toxic. Tender swelling on limb. Septic arthritis.
Investigation. Culture blood and aspirate from the infection site.
Treatment.
- Intravenous antibiotics for 7 days then oral for five weeks.
- Immobilisation and analgesics for pain relief.
- Surgical drainage if symptoms present for more than 72 hours.
Prognosis. Epiphyseal damage in infants can affect growth. 5% develop chronic osteomyelitis.

JOINT PAINS
Commonly:
- Acute trauma. ? Non-accidental injury.
- Chronic trauma: chondromalacia patellae.
- Transient viral arthritis.
- Irritable hip syndrome.

Less commonly:
- Septic arthritis.
- Juvenile chronic arthritis.
- Reactive arthritis.
- Henoch-Schönlein purpura.
- Osteochondritis.
- Slipped epiphysis (head of femur).
- Congenital dislocation of the hip.

Rarely:
- Metabolic: gout, scurvy, rickets.
- Neoplastia (osteosarcoma, nephroblastoma, leukaemia).
- Collagen disorders (SLE).
- Enteropathic arthritis (Crohn's, ulcerative colitis).
- Allergy (food, drugs).
- Blood disorders (haemophilia, sickle-cell, thalassaemia)

Investigation of arthritis.
- Microscopy and culture synovial fluid, blood culture (? sepsis).
- FBC and differential, ESR.
- X-ray affected joints.
- Clotting times and factor analysis (if haemarthrosis).
- Stool culture (? if recent diarrhoea).

Additional investigations for chronic arthritis.
- Blood for Hb, urate, anti-nuclear antibody, anti-double stranded DNA, rheumatoid factor, ASOT, viral titres.
- Bone marrow aspiration (if marked systemic upset).

Transient viral arthritis
Incidence. Common. Follows erythema infectiosum (parvovirus type 19) > rubella > mumps, chickenpox, infectious mononucleosis, viral hepatitis.
Clinically. A mild migratory polyarthritis affecting the hands and knees. Spontaneous resolution without residual arthritis.

Irritable hip
Incidence. Commonest hip pain in children. Boys > girls. Age 4 to 10.

Aetiology. Transient synovitis.
Clinically. Hip pain and limp.
Investigation. A diagnosis of exclusion, X-ray of both hips and femurs should be normal. Normal FBC and ESR.
Prognosis. 90% settle within 7 days on bed rest and paracetamol. 15% recur, usually within a year. No residual defect.

Slipped upper femoral epiphysis
Uncommon. Age 10 to 20. Gradually increasing pain in hip. Restricted abduction. X-ray is diagnostic. Requires surgical correction. Avascular necrosis of the epiphysis is the commonest complication.

Hypermobility syndrome
Incidence. Common, girls > boys. Familial.
Clinically. Joint (knee) pains after exertion. Three or more of the following signs of ligamentous laxity:
- Thumb can be pushed back to touch the anterior surface of forearm.
- 5th metacarpophalangeal joint flexes to 90%.
- Elbow hyperextends by 10° or more.
- Knee hyperextends by 10° or more.
- Can put palms on floor with knees extended.

Management. Avoid exercises that cause pain.
Prognosis. Hypermobility reduces with age. In severe cases osteoarthritis develops (Marfan's syndrome, Ehlers Danlos syndrome, osteogenesis imperfecta).

Chondromalacia patella
Incidence. Common in adolescence. Girls > boys.
Pathology. Degeneration of the cartilage.
Clinically. Knee pains that are worse when coming down stairs and after sitting down. Pressing on the patella causes pain. Palpable crepitus on moving the knee joint.
Investigation. X–rays are usually normal, but the 'skyline' view of the knee is the first to suggest thinning of the cartilage.
Treatment. Rest when painful. Analgesics. Soft tissue surgery to alter the dynamics of the joint. Patellectomy is the last resort.
Prognosis. Usually resolves by age 30.

Septic arthritis
Incidence. Uncommon. 50% are younger than 4 years old.

Aetiology. Usually Staphylococcus aureus. Under age 4 Haemophilus influenzae is also common. Pneumococcus in infants and immunocompromised children. Gonococcus in sexually active adolescents or sexually abused children. Tuberculous arthritis is rare in the UK.

Clinically. Usually monoarthritis (80% affect weight bearing joints - hips, knees, ankles). Gonococcus and meningococcus can cause a peripheral migratory polyarthritis.

Management. Isolate the organism by culturing blood and synovial fluid. Splint the joint in the position of rest until acute inflammation settles. Antibiotics intravenously for 48 hours or until clinical improvement. Analgesics. Surgical drainage if the hip is affected or if no better after 4 days.

Prognosis. Good result if treatment is started within 48 hours of onset or if infection is gonococcal. Permanent arthritis follows in 40% of infected hip joints, 30% of ankles, 10% of knees.

Reactive arthritis

Incidence. Rare, 90% carry HLA B27.

Aetiology. Usually follows enteritis (Salmonella, Shigella, Yersinia, Campylobacter). May follow Chlamydia infection in sexually active adolescents. Rheumatic fever is rare in the UK. Lyme disease is increasingly diagnosed.

Clinically. Onset within 10 days of the infection. Usually lower limb oligoarthritis. Enthesopathy. Iritis. In Reiter's syndrome there is also one or more of: urethritis, conjunctivitis, oral ulceration, keratoderma blenorrhagica.

Investigation. High WBC and ESR.

Treatment. Indomethacin. Steroid injections for refractory joints or entheses.

Prognosis. Usually settles in 1 to 12 months. May recur following further bowel infections. Up to 10% develop disabling arthritis.

Juvenile chronic arthritis (JCA)

Arthritis lasting more than 3 months with no identified cause.

Incidence. 1/1,000 children develop JCA at some time. Commonly age 2-4. Girls > boys. May be familial (ankylosing spondylitis, psoriatic arthritis).

Clinically. Joints are stiff, painful and swollen.

10% Still's disease.

- Age 1 to 5. Girls = boys.
- Starts with systemic symptoms: malaise, high fever at night, maculopapular erythematous rash on the limbs, lymphadenopathy, hepato-splenomegaly, pericarditis. Systemic symptoms last for up to 6 months.

- A chronic destructive polyarthritis starts during the systemic symptoms. Affects knees, wrists, carpi, ankles and tarsi. 25% have progressive arthritis.
- Increased ESR and circulating polymorphonuclear lymphocytes.

30% Polyarticular (Rheumatoid Factor Negative).
- Age 1 to 16. 90% girls.
- Starts with polyarthritis (knees, wrists, ankles). Flexor tenosynovitis. 10% have progressive arthritis with early fusion of the epiphyses of affected joints (cervical apophyseal joints and temporomandibular joints (small jaw)).
- Systemic symptoms are mild. Chronic iridocyclitis in the 25% with anti-nuclear antibody (ANA). Some develop psoriasis or inflammatory bowel disease.

10% Polyarticular (Rheumatoid Factor Positive).
- Age 8 to 16. 85% girls.
- Starts with polyarthritis (interphalangeal joints). Rheumatoid nodules and vasculitis. 50% develop progressive arthritis, by age 15 years about one third are severely disabled.
- Systemic symptoms may be severe.

35% Pauciarticular with onset in early childhood.
- Up to 4 joints mildly affected (knee, ankle, elbow). Progressive arthritis uncommon.
- Few systemic symptoms. 50% have chronic iridocyclitis (ANA positive).

15% Pauciarticular with onset in late childhood (juvenile ankylosing spondylitis).
- 90% boys with HLAB27.
- Up to 4 joints affected (hip, knee). Sacroiliitis, enthesopathy and ankylosing spondylosis common but of variable severity. One third develop severe arthritis of the hips. Progressive arthritis uncommon. Gold or penicillamine do not help.
- Acute iridocyclitis in 25%.

Progressive arthritis may occur with any variant - anaemia, growth retardation, amyloidosis with proteinuria.

Treatment of acute arthritis.
Aspirin, indomethacin or ibuprofen.
Prednisolone orally for severe systemic symptoms.
Encourage activity and avoid bed rest if possible. Passive physiotherapy and splinting to maintain function in affected joints. Active physiotherapy, especially swimming, once pain controlled.

Treatment of severe progressive arthritis.
- Gold injections, penicillamine or chloroquine may be needed for years. Azathioprine for resistant cases.
- Mechanical and electronic aids including wheelchairs.
- Special educational provisions.
- Ophthalmic review at least yearly if ANA positive (?iridocyclitis).

Prognosis. About 5% die in childhood with infection or amyloidosis. On reaching adult life: 60% are normal, 20% have mild disability and 20% are moderately or severely disabled.

OSTEOCHONDRITIS

Idiopathic avascular necrosis of an ossification centre which collapses. Repair occurs around ingrowing capillaries.
- **Osgood Schlatter's disease** of the tibial tubercle is common.
- **Perthes' disease** of the femoral head.
- **Scheuermann's disease** of the vertebral ring epiphyses.
- **Calve's disease** of the vertebral body.

Perthes' disease

Incidence. Affects 1/2000 children at any one time. Boys (80%). Age 4 to 9 years. Bilateral in 15%. Associated with familial retinoblastoma.

Clinically. Hip pain and limp.

Management. Diagnosis by X-ray (changes may only show months after the onset of pain). Prevent subluxation of the femoral head by bed rest with traction in abduction. Femoral osteotomy if traction fails. Definitive surgery, including hip replacement, once the disease is inactive.

Prognosis. In adult life 80% are normal or have minor symptoms, of the 20% with hip pain a quarter require hip replacement. Significant arthritis in 0% with onset before age 5, 40% with onset aged 6 to 9, 100% with onset after age 9.

SPACE OCCUPYING LESIONS IN BONE
- **Bone cysts.**
- **Benign neoplasm:** osteoid osteoma, chondroma.
- **Malignant neoplasm: osteosarcoma, secondary neoplasm.**
- **Abscess.**
- **Granuloma:** TB syphilis, non-infective.
- **Fibrous dysplasia.**

Bone cysts

Asymptomatic unless bone fractures. Affects long bones. X-ray reveals a circumscribed translucent area with no surrounding sclerosis. Large cysts can be curetted and packed with bone chips.

Osteoid osteoma

Schoolage boys > girls. X-ray: translucent lesion with surrounding sclerosis. Pain at night relieved by aspirin. Benign. Excise.

Chondroma

Proliferations of cartilage in or on bones, especially in the hands or feet. Present as painless, swellings, fractures or disturbed epiphyseal growth. 10% become malignant (chondrosarcoma). Excise.

Osteochondroma

Commonest benign tumour of bone. A nest of cartilage cells left behind by a growing epiphyseal plate. Forms a cartilage cap on a calcified stalk attached to the main bone. Often stops growing after puberty. May interfere with epiphyseal growth. 1% become malignant. Excise.

Osteosarcoma

Incidence. 200 cases per year in the UK, 70% children. Boys > girls.
Pathology. Sited in the metaphysis of a long bone (lower femur > upper tibia >> upper femur, humerus). At diagnosis 20% have gross metastases and 80% have micrometastases.
Clinically. Painful swelling.
Diagnosis. X-ray - osteolytic or osteosclerotic. CxR and bone scan for gross metastases.
Treatment. Palliative amputation for advanced local disease. Local excision for small lesions. Excision of pulmonary metastases. Chemotherapy increases survival but the optimum regime has not been established.
Prognosis. Long term survival is 70% overall (but only 10% for those with gross metastases on diagnosis). Relapses after surgery and chemotherapy are usually pulmonary (80%) and occur within 2 years.

Polyostotic fibrous dysplasia

Parts of bones are replaced by masses of fibrous tissue. Presents in childhood with swellings in bones which bend and fracture.

CONGENITAL DEFORMITIES

Congenital dislocation of the hip (CDH)
Incidence. Unstable hips are found in 1% of neonates screened. 0.2% of neonates with clinically normal hips will later develop CDH. At risk: female (70%), breech delivery, family history, caucasian, muscle weakness.
Clinically. Hips are dislocated or can be dislocated easily. Late walker.
Investigation. ultrasound > X-ray.
Treatment. Splint neonates in abduction (Aberdeen splint for 6 weeks or Von Rosen splint for 12 weeks), reduction by serial splinting or abduction traction in late-diagnosed cases. Surgery if conservative methods fail: adductor tenotomy, open reduction, femoral osteotomy, acetabular reconstruction.
Prognosis. 90% of neonates with unstable hips become normal without treatment. 1% of those requiring splints will require surgery. Cases diagnosed after 6 months show an increasing incidence of premature osteoarthritis, avascular necrosis and pseudoarthrosis.

Genu recurvatum = hyperextension at the knee.
• Mild. Common in infancy but better by early childhood.
• Severe, congenital. Associated with congenital dislocation of the hips, club foot, hypermobility syndrome, cerebral palsy. Tendency to backward dislocation. Treat with splints and braces to restrict extension, and muscle building exercises to support the knee. Occasionally osteotomies are needed.
• Severe, acquired. Joint damage.

Bow knees (genu varum)
• Physiological bow knees. Normal up to age 3, when it resolves spontaneously. When the medial malleoli are together the knees are symetrically separated by less than 5 cm.
• Pathological bow knees are usually associated with tibial torsion and treated by tibial osteotomy.

Knock knees (genu valgum)
• Physiological knock knees. Normal from age 3 to 5 years, when it resolves spontaneously. With the thighs together the medial malleoli are symetrically separated by less than 10 cm apart.
• Pathological knock knees are associated with flat feet, obesity and a family history of severe knock knees. Staple the medial femoral or tibial epiphysis by age 12 or perform a supracondylar osteotomy after epiphyseal closure.

TOES TURNED IN
- Metatarsus varus. Hooked forefoot but normal heel. Full passive dorsiflexion and eversion. Normal gait. Better by 4 years old.
- Club foot.
- Medial tibial torsion. The tibia is bowed laterally and twisted so that the feet are turned in when the patellae are pointing forwards. Better by age 5.
- Anteversion of the femoral neck. When the patellae faces forward the femoral neck is externally rotated. The child is more comfortable with the toes turned in.

Club foot (talipes equino-varus)
Incidence. 1/1000 live births. Male (60%). Bilateral in 50%.
Aetiology. Usually primary sporadic. Occasionally primary familial (10% recurrence in siblings). Sometimes secondary to neuromuscular disorders (spina bifida, cerebral palsy) or bony abnormalities (congenital vertical talus).
Clinically. Neonate. The sole of the foot is rotated medially and plantar flexed. The foot cannot be pushed passively into full dorsiflexion and eversion. The calf and peroneal muscles, and the soft tissues of the medial side of the foot, are shortened and underdeveloped. The heel is high (poorly formed). Eventually the tarsal bones become deformed stabilising the deformity.
Management. Adhesive strapping to hold the foot in eversion and dorsiflexion. Parents should manually overcorrect the deformity several times each day. At 3 months of age, if the deformity is improving, prescribe Dennis Browne boots with a crossbar splint until age 1 year. If the deformity is not improving do soft tissue releases then prescribe boots. Surgical boots once walking. Severe or neglected cases need osteotomies.

Flat foot (pes planus)
Incidence. Physiological up to age 3, but commonly persists. Severe deformities are usually secondary to muscle weakness (spina bifida, muscular dystrophy).
Clinically. The medial longitudinal arch is flat. Adults may present with foot strain but children are presented by parents who have noted the cosmetic defect or excessive wear on the medial surface of the shoe heel.
Management. A wedge (base medially) under the heel evens out shoe wear. Exercises to strengthen the intrinsic foot flexors have a placebo effect. Arthrodesis is reserved for severe deformities or adults with intractable pain.

Claw foot (pes cavus)
Uncommon. Usually idiopathic (may be autosomal dominant). Sometimes secondary to muscular imbalance (spina bifida). Examination reveals a high arched foot, prominent metatarsal heads, clawed toes. Advise the parents on exercises to keep the foot supple. May need metatarsal pads, soft tissue releases, tendon transplants, osteotomies and arthrodeses.

TOE DEFORMITIES
- Mallet toe: hyperflexed at the distal interphalangeal joint.
- Hammer toe: hyperflexed at the proximal interphalangeal joint.
- Claw toe: hyperflexed at both interphalangeal joints.
- Curly toes.

Management. May be isolated or part of a complex defect. Isolated toe deformities usually resolve by age 3 with sensible, broad ended, shoes. Soft tissue releases or arthrodesis are occasionally necessary.

SCOLIOSIS
Lateral curvature of the spine. Affects 4% of children.
Postural scoliosis: disappears when the spine is flexed. Usually idiopathic or compensatory for a short leg. Occasionally pain relieving or hysterical. It does not progress.
Structural scoliosis: does not correct on flexion. Vertebrae are rotated with their spines indicating the concavity of the curve and a 'rib-hump' on the convexity.
- 2.5% Idiopathic infantile scoliosis: Age 0-3 years. Usually males with plagiocephaly. 90% resolve within 3 years.
- 2.5% Idiopathic juvenile scoliosis: Age 4-9 years. Features of both infantile and adolescent scoliosis.
- 60% Idiopathic adolescent scoliosis: Age 10-15 years. Girls > boys. Presents with deformity. Pain is unusual until adult life. Progression may be halted by exercises and spinal brace. Serial plaster casts, halo-pelvic traction and spinal fusion may be needed. Severe kyphoscoliosis may cause hypoventilation and cor pulmonale.
- 35% are secondary to abnormal vertebrae (congenitally abnormal, damaged or diseased) or muscle imbalance (spina bifida or cerebral palsy).

METABOLIC AND HEREDITARY BONE DISEASES

Osteogenesis imperfecta (brittle bone disease)
Incidence. 1/10,000 live births.
Pathology. There is a defect in collagen. Diaphyses of long bones are thin.
Clinically. The severe form is not familial: frequent fractures in infancy heal with progressive deformity and death in childhood, dental defects. The mild form is an autosomal dominant: occasional fractures starting in childhood or adolescence, blue sclerae, adults become deaf (otosclerosis). No specific therapy.

Osteopetrosis (marble bone disease)
Pathology. Defective bone remodelling by osteoclasts. Bones are thicker but weaker. The marrow is replaced by bone.
Clinically.
* The severe form is autosomal recessive, presents with neonatal fractures and results in childhood death as a result of fractures or marrow failure.
* The mild form (80%) is autosomal dominant and presents with frequent fractures in childhood, scoliosis (20%) or nerve compression syndromes (deafness in 50%). No specific treatment.

Achondroplasia.
Pathology. Commonest skeletal dysplasia. Autosomal dominant, but 90% are new mutations (commoner with old fathers). Reduced formation of bone in cartilage (long bones, base of skull).
Clinically. The neonate is small and mildly hypotonic. Limbs are bowed with bulbous bone ends. Fingers are all the same length (trident hand). Small face, frontal bossing, depressed nasal bridge. Intelligence is normal unless affected by hydrocephalus which is common. Some affected children develop cord compression syndrome. Adults are fertile with no progressive deformity and a normal life expectancy. No particular susceptibility to arthritis.

Marfan's syndrome
Incidence. Autosomal dominant. 3 per 200,000 live births.
Clinically.
* Long fingers and limbs (like Abraham Lincoln), hypermobile joints, high arched palate, dislocated lens, adolescent scoliosis (50%).
* Cardiovascular defects kill by age 50: thoracic aortic aneurysm, aortic and mitral valve incompetence.
Infertile.

25. ONCOLOGY

EPIDEMIOLOGY
Malignant diseases occur in 1 in 10,000 children each year. 1 child in 600 will
develop a malignancy. The average GP will see 1 new case in 20 years.
Although malignancies are rare they are the second commonest cause of death
in schoolchildren.

40%   Reticuloendothelial tumours: leukaemia, lymphoma.
22%   Central nervous system tumours: 70% occur below the tentorium.
26%   Embryonic mesenchymal tumours: nephroblastoma.
2%   Germ cell tumours.
10%   Others.

There are occasionally recognised risk factors:
- Chromosomal abnormalities: Down's syndrome and acute lymphoblastic
  leukaemia.
- Single gene abnormalities: polyposis coli and adenocarcinoma, neuro-
  fibromatosis and sarcomas, retinoblastoma.
- Intrauterine radiation exposure in the first trimester.

MANAGEMENT
See chapter 48 of 'Child Care in General Practice' for further details.
1. Medical and nursing staff must keep the family informed (with consistent
   information) and allow discussion about:
   - The diagnosis. Prognosis for the patient. Risk of siblings being affected.
   - Advice on daily care: diet, activity, education, immunisation including
     immunoglobulin injections after exposure to infectious diseases.
   - The response to warning signs such as fever and weight loss.
   - Treatment options and their side effects: immune supression (infections),
     growth retardation, sterility, damage to endocrine glands (diabetes), and
     new malignancy.
2. Referral to other professionals (teachers, social workers), support groups,
   charities and government organisations.
3. Depression, anxiety and behaviour problems affecting the patient or his
   family will need appropriate care.
4. Bereavement.
   - A family can grieve for a dying child then find it difficult to cope with
     the news that the child is cured.
   - A family may have completed grieving during a prolonged illness and
     then experience guilt at feeling relieved when the child eventually dies.
   - The fear that siblings will also be affected complicates the bereavement
     process.

26. THE EXAMINATION

THE LONDON EXAMINATION

THE SYLLABUS
The DCH tests **primary care** paediatrics:
(a) The epidemiology, prevention, diagnosis and management of common and important disorders of childhood. Chronic handicap.
(b) Health promotion:
- Pre- and perinatal care as it affects the subsequent progress of the infant. Genetic counselling. Preparation for parenthood. The care of the normal newborn.
- Normal physical, mental and emotional growth. Health surveillance. The management of minor abnormalities.
- Health promotion by education, immunisation and screening. Feeding and nutrition. Social aspects of child health.
- Social agencies and the law affecting children.
- Education.

EXAMINATION FORMAT
Paper 1
- **10 short note questions.** Worth 50% of the marks for this paper. Each question should be about 100 words long and take 9 minutes to answer (Allow 90 minutes for this section).
- **2 Case commentaries.** These are presented as 100-300 word stories followed by 3-5 questions. Allow 45 minutes for each commentary which is worth 25% of the marks for this paper.

Paper II
60 multiple choice questions (MCQs) in 2 hours. Each question is presented as a 'stem' statement followed by 5 parts. You can answer true or false to each part by marking an answer paper. Unanswered questions score 0, but wrong answers score -1. You must pass paper II in order to attend for the clinical examination.

Clinical
- **The long case** consists of 40 minutes spent with the patient and 20 minutes discussing the case with the examiners.
- **The short cases** test your ability to examine children of various ages and recognize abnormalities. About 10 minutes are spent with developmental assessments and testing the special senses. Another 15 minutes are devoted to children with physical signs.

HINTS
Short notes
Answer only the question in front of you. Do not write down *everything* you know about the subject mentioned. Do not spend longer than 9 minutes on answers about which you know more, because you need to allow thinking time for the questions you find difficult.

Try to convey one relevant fact or concept with every 5 words. Each relevant fact scores a mark. I have two standard frameworks on which I base answers, but every answer does not use the whole of a framework.

Question "Discuss condition X"
- **Definition and range of severity.**
- **Incidence**: ? common, ? age, ? male, ? social class V, ? urban.
- **Pathology**: gross, microscopic, biochemical, genetic.
- **Cause**: TIN CAN BED PAN = Trauma, infection, neoplasm, collagen, allergic (and drug reaction), neurological, blood, endocrine, developmental, psychiatric, arterial (and venous), normal variation.
- **Symptoms and signs.**
- **Differential diagnosis** starting with the commonest.
- **Investigations** (divided into those arranged by a GP and those arranged by a specialist).
- **Treatment**: treat the family not just the child.
  - Prevention: pre-conception (genetic counselling), antenatal care, antenatal diagnosis and selective abortion, intra-partum care, diet and lifestyle, immunisation, screening for abnormalities.
  - Advice.
  - Medication.
  - Special education,
  - Referral: social worker, psychologist or psychiatrist, physiotherapist, occupational therapist (provision of aids and prostheses), surgeon.
- **Prognosis.**

Question "What would you say to the parents of a child with condition X?"
- What do you know about your child's illness?
- What do you think caused it?
- How does it affect your child?
- How does it affect the rest of the family?
- My knowledge of this condition as it affects your child is....
- The risk that other members of the family will be affected is....

- The possible treatments are....
- The other professionals I wish to involve are....
- The progress I expect is....
- Further information can be obtained from....
- Please let me see you and your child on....

Case commentaries

These questions assess your approach to psycho-social problems and the continuing care of chronic illness. Think widely when answering these questions. If you concentrate on the clinical problem you will miss easy marks. There are certain underlying themes that you are expected to be familiar with:

- The options for health promotion starting with pre-conception counselling and ending with sex-education for adolescents.
- The role of health visitors, district nurses, social workers, teachers and the school health service.
- The role of voluntary organisations and self-help groups.
- The relevant legislation.
- Respect for a child's wishes with appropriate regard for their age.
- The influence of social class and race on the pattern of disease and the response to medical care.
- The diagnosis and management of child abuse. This includes neglect, emotional abuse, physical abuse and sexual abuse.
- Nutrition.
- The care of the child **and** his family ought to be part of every answer. It is particularly important when the child is dying, chronically sick or handicapped. Remember that a child often has siblings as well as parents.
- The interaction between the doctor, the patient and his parents. The effect of this relationship on the presentation of problems and the response to therapy.

We recommend 'Child Care in General Practice' as background reading for these topics.

Multiple choice questions

You must develop your own approach to these by doing lots of MCQs. My approach (JB) is to start at number 1 and mark the answers I am sure of. When I reach the end I count how many I have marked and how many more I have to answer in order to pass. I then go back and mark the answers I am reasonably sure of until I have answered sufficient questions. Wild guesses are heavily penalised by the negative marking of incorrect answers.

The Clinical

The only way to pass the clinical is to examine lots of children under the tuition of an expert. Unless you see lots of children you cannot develop a pattern of examination or learn how to get children to cooperate. You need tuition in order to develop good habits.

- **The long case** tests your ability to take and present a history including social, behavioural and educational aspects. A good way to develop your technique is to present cases to a paediatric consultant or a colleague who has passed the DCH. You may not enjoy exposing yourself to such scrutiny but failing the examination is also uncomfortable.

- **Short cases.** Become competent at the things a General Practitioner or Clinical Medical Officer should know. You will be expected to be able to distinguish an innocent flow murmur from aortic valve stenosis, but you will be forgiven for missing reversed splitting of the second heart sound. You must be fluent in the various techniques of developmental surveillance. When you apply to take the DCH, the Royal College of Physicians will send you detailed guidelines on the assessment of vision and hearing. It is unwise to ignore their advice.

THE GLASGOW EXAMINATION

The syllabus is broadly similar to that of the London Examination, but the examination has a different format.

Paper 1. Principles of Child Health.

Paper II. The Practice of Paediatrics.

Clinical examination.

Oral examination.

INDEX

PASTEST REVISION BOOKS

PasTest are specialists in Postgraduate Medical Education. Our revision book and practice examinations are written by medical experts and Royal College examiners. PasTest publications are available for the following examinations:

MRCP Part 1 Adult Medicine & Paediatrics
MRCP Part 2 Adult Medicine & Paediatrics
MRCGP   DRCOG
MRCOG   DCH
FRCS   FRCA
PLAB

Please contact us by post, telephone or fax for full details of our books and a price list. All orders are despatched on the same day they are received. We accept Access, Visa and Switch cards.

PASTEST INTENSIVE REVISION COURSES

MRCP Part 1 Adult Medicine   MRCP Part 1 Paediatrics
MRCP Part 2 Adult Medicine   MRCP Part 2 Paediatrics
MRCP Part 2 Clinicals   MRCGP
DRCOG   DCH
PLAB

PasTest Intensive Revision Courses are available for each of the above examinations. All the courses stress successful exam technique and all course material is based on past Royal College questions. All PasTest lecturers are experienced and enthusiastic experts. Courses are held at convenient centres in London and Manchester, and are approved under HM63/27, Section 63 or PGEA.

For full details about PasTest books and courses please telephone, fax or write to us today.

**PasTest, FREEPOST, Rankin House, Parkgate Estate,
Knutsford, Cheshire WA16 7BR
Telephone 0565 755226   Fax 0565 650264**